S0-CFA-161

an introduction to

HOLISTIC HERBS

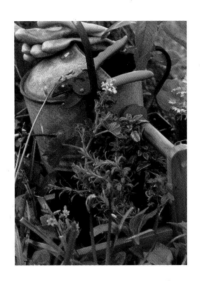

p

an introduction to

HOLISTIC HERBS

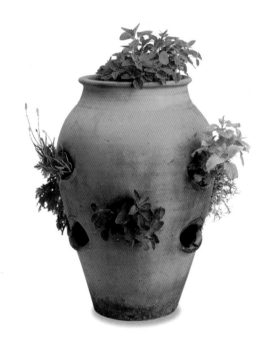

Jennie Harding

This is a Parragon Publishing book
First published in 2002

Parragon Publishing
Queen Street House
4 Queen Street
Bath BA1 1HE

Copyright © Exclusive Editions 2002

All rights reserved. No part of this publication may be
reproduced, stored in a retrieval system, or transmitted
in any form or by any means, electronic, mechanical,
photocopying, recording, or otherwise, without the
prior written permission of the copyright owner.

This book was created by
THE BRIDGEWATER BOOK COMPANY

Art director *Stephen Knowlden*
Designers *Chris and Jane Lanaway*
Editorial director *Fiona Biggs*
Project editor *Lizzy Gray*
Picture researcher *Trudi Valter*

ISBN 1-84273-440-7

Manufactured in China

Contents

Introduction   6

What is a **herb?**   8

Ancient **herbal history**   10

Famous **herbalists**   12

Herbs in **modern times**   14

Herbs in your **environment**   16

Growing herbs   18

Sunny spaces and **shady places**   20

Beautiful by design   22

Miniature **herb** garden   24

Herbs in the **wild**   28

A–Z of **herbs**   29

Making herbal preparations   70

Natural **skin** and **hair** care   74

Herbs for general **health care**   76

Herbs to **relieve stress**   78

First aid with herbs   80

Herbs in the **kitchen**   82

Herbal **recipes to enjoy**   84

Herbs **around** the **home**   86

A medical herbalist—
meet Kelly Holden   88

Receiving treatment
with herbal medicine   90

Glossary   92

Useful addresses   94

Index   95

Introduction

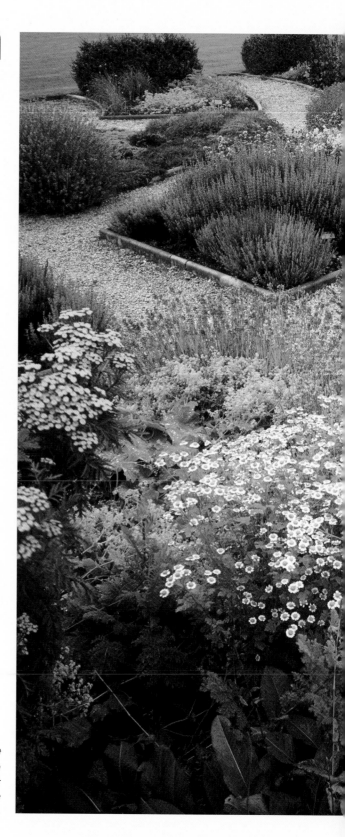

Welcome to *Holistic Herbs*—and the start of a journey. We start with a look back through history, discovering that herbs have served humankind as flavorings and medicines for thousands of years. Further on, many creative suggestions will show how herbs can improve your environment. You will discover 40 different herbs, learning how to grow them yourself and how to use them. Along the way, there will be surprises—you may well find that herbs you have been using for a long time have other unexpected properties.

Herbs have been used in cookery and medicine throughout the centuries.

The aim of this book is to encourage you to reconnect with the natural world through growing and using herbs. Many of the plants featured in the text are still found growing wild in locations where they originated, and have been part of food and medicine in those regions for a very long time. You probably know many of them already and are used to obtaining them from supermarkets or

Cultivating a herb garden is very rewarding: it will provide you with your own stock of fresh herbs, which you can use in cooking and for medicinal purposes. You can also enjoy the garden as an area for relaxation and leisure.

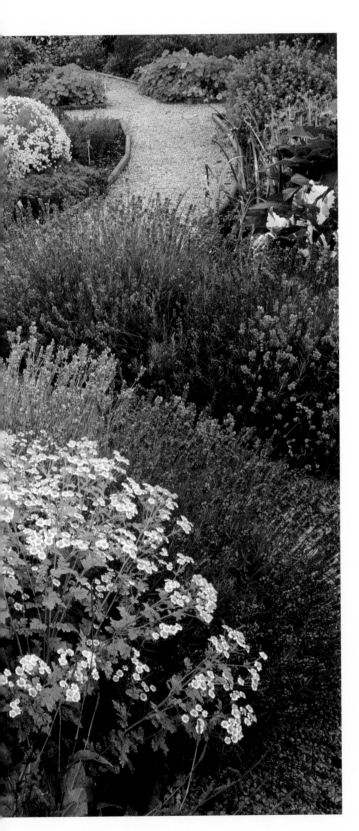

health food shops, yet you may wonder—how do they look and smell as plants? It can be fun and rewarding to find out. There is no substitute for fresh herbs you have produced yourself—the flavors and fragrances are such a pleasure to experience, and the taste is far superior to dried or frozen. As you will discover, you do not need to have a garden— balconies, yards, even windowsills can be used and transformed into herbal havens.

Even in the mad rush of modern life, your sense of smell can still be beguiled, making you stop and inhale the fragrances of herbs in a sun-warmed garden. Aromatic herbs have a long history of use as mental and emotional de-stressors; throughout history Ancient Greek physicians, Arab doctors, Benedictine monks, and country housewives have all valued herbs as tonics to the spirit as well as to the body. By creating your own space to grow herbs, you are participating in an activity that will connect you to ancient wisdom.

Enjoy this book, and may you create your own herbal haven as a source of delight in your life!

You can also grow fresh herbs in planters and pots on a balcony, terrace, or patio area.

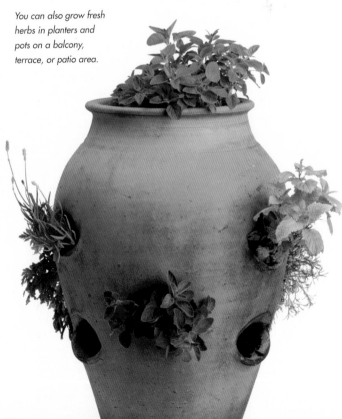

What is a **herb?**

All herbs are plants, but not all plants are herbs. Humankind has always used plants for shelter, clothing, food, medicine, dyes, and more; yet herbs remain special, in a class of their own. The word "herb" comes from the Latin *herba*, meaning "grass" or "green plants"; yet herbs were in use long before Roman times. The Chinese text *The Yellow Emperor's Book of Internal Medicine* dates back to approximately 2000 BCE and mentions plants such as ginger as an aromatic spice and medicinal remedy.

CHILES

For thousands of years before civilization, human beings wandered the planet in tribes and groups. Together with hunting, the gathering of edible plants was an important activity and often vital to survival. It is likely that our distant ancestors discovered and used certain plants as foods and medicines by directly smelling, tasting, and chewing them; even today, jungle survival techniques for "testing" a plant involve trying it out several times, each time observing any sensations, then eventually swallowing it, exactly as the hunter-gatherers must have done thousands of years ago.

Today, many of us immediately think of herbs as flavorings for cooking, and there is an ever-rising interest in different styles of food preparation from around the world. Tastes and aromas define a culture; the tomato, thyme, and oregano tastes of Mediterranean dishes contrast with the lemongrass, chile and coconut zest of Thai recipes. People are now enjoying herbs and spices in the kitchen more than ever before. The aromas of herbs and spices are literally "mouth-watering," as they encourage the body to produce digestive juices to assist the breakdown of food.

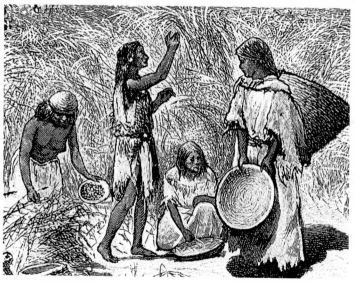

People are now enjoying a wider range of flavors from around the world, such as coconut combined with lemongrass and chile for a taste of Thai cookery.

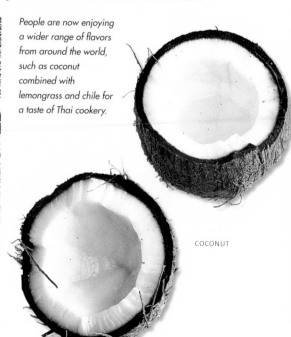

COCONUT

Yet many of those kitchen ingredients are also important medicinal remedies within the herbalist's kit, being used slightly differently to help in the prevention or treatment of illness. The boundary between the kitchen and the medicine chest is often quite hazy. Herbs have been with us as both flavorings and remedies for a very long time and this is why they are special.

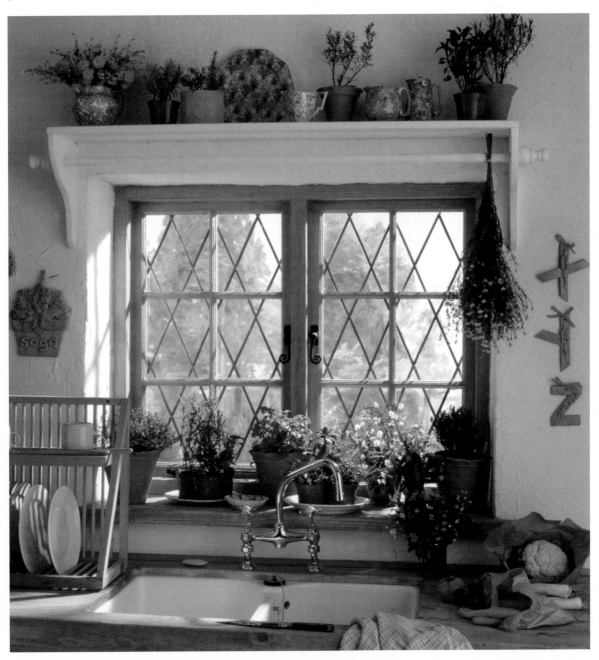

You can also grow fresh herbs in pots on a shelf or windowsill in your kitchen. This makes them readily accessible for adding to dishes and also provides a handy space for growing them if you have not got a garden or your garden is overcrowded.

Ancient **herbal history**

Ancient documents and archaeological evidence tell of herbs and spices still used today. Sacred Indian Vedic texts more than 2,000 years old mention an extensive range of aromatic ingredients, such as coriander and sandalwood, which were used to worship the gods and heal the sick. The tomb of the boy pharaoh Tutankhamun yielded not just jewels, but also a wealth of botanical evidence of herbs, spices, resins, and plants, such as frankincense, fenugreek, thyme, or garlic, which were part of everyday life in ancient Egyptian times.

FRANKINCENSE

The roots of Western herbal medicine lie with the ancient Greeks. The physician Hippocrates (460–377 BCE) evolved an approach to healing based on the elements earth, air, fire, and water, and the corresponding aspects of the human body—blood, phlegm, yellow, and black bile. Hippocrates used herbs as one element of his approach to disease, which he understood to be an imbalance of these "humours." Pedanius Dioscorides (c. 40-90 CE), a military physician serving the Roman emperor Nero, wrote a five-volume work *De Materia Medica*, a major catalog of the medicinal plants of the Mediterranean, which served as a reference work for 1,500 years.

In the early medieval Arab culture, Abu Ali Sina (980–1037 CE), known as Avicenna, was an astonishing individual skilled in astronomy, geometry, metaphysics, medicine, and much more. His *Canon of Medicine* cataloged 811 known medicinal substances, including herbs of Chinese, Tibetan, and Indian origin, showing how far these aromatic herbs traveled even at that time. He is credited with developing a form of distillation used to extract essential oils from aromatic plants.

This medieval image of the Four Humors depicts the qualities in human form.

Many herbs, spices, resins, and plants, such as frankincense, fenugreek, thyme, and garlic, were found in the tomb of Tutankhamun.

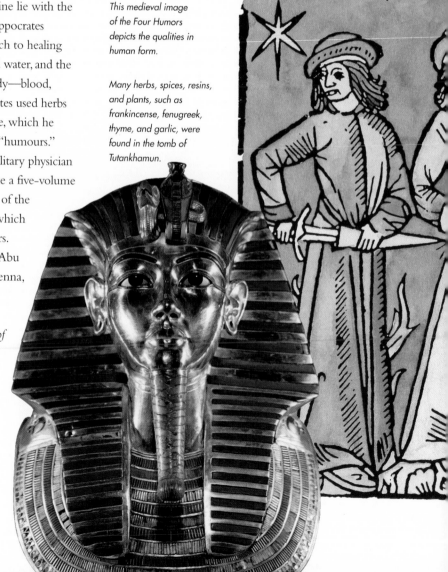

In the 12th century, the German prophetess, abbess, mystic, and healer Hildegard of Bingen (1098-1179 CE) wrote several works on the healing properties of herbs, encouraging their use medicinally and in food. She also regarded the properties of plants as spiritual links to the Creator, embodying the quality of *viriditas,* or "greening," which today we might call life force. Her healing methods are used in Southern Germany today, where her recipe for bread made with spelt flour (*Triticum spelta*) is still eaten to promote vitality.

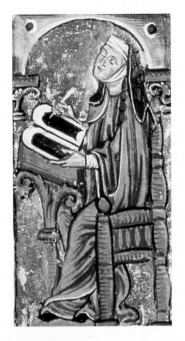

At the "Hildegard Practice" in Konstanz in Germany, the teachings of Hildegard of Bingen are still followed and used for treating patients. A naturopathic approach to healing based on diet, rest, and rebalancing the four humors is taken. Health and well-being are established on all three levels—physical, mental, and spiritual.

The German mystic, prophetess, and healer Hildegard of Bingen (1098–1179 CE) supported the use of herbs in medicine and cookery. She wrote several works on the subject.

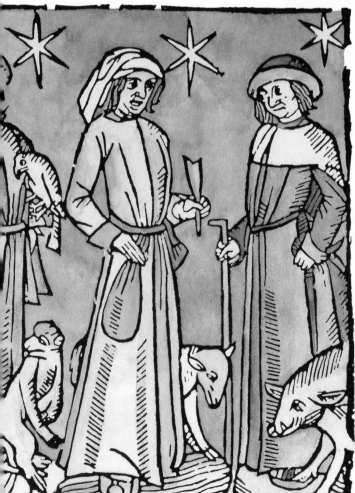

FOUR HUMORS

This system explained mental and physical health as an interplay of four elemental fluids, or "humors" which gave rise to a person's mental and physical characteristics. The humors were said to rise to the brain, and any imbalance in the four was said to explain a person's mental or physical state. Excess humors were "related" by bloodletting, either by opening a vein with a knife or by applying leeches.

BLOOD: related to the Air element, with hot and moist properties, giving an amorous, happy, and generous nature called SANGUINE

YELLOW BILE: related to the Fire element, with hot and dry properties, giving a violent and vengeful nature called CHOLERIC

PHLEGM: related to the Water element, with cold and moist properties, giving a dull, pale, and cowardly nature called PHLEGMATIC

BLACK BILE: related to the Earth element, with cold and dry properties, giving a gluttonous, lazy, and sentimental nature called MELANCHOLIC

GARLIC

Famous **herbalists**

The golden age of English herbalism spanned the 16th and 17th centuries. The lives of these herbalists were highly influential and their work continues to influence Western herbal medicine today. Their books helped to spread information about the uses of herbs and also condensed existing knowledge into a format that survived the rise of drug-based medicine. Nicholas Culpeper in particular has become a household name, and his book *Culpeper's Complete Herbal* can still be found in many kitchens nowadays.

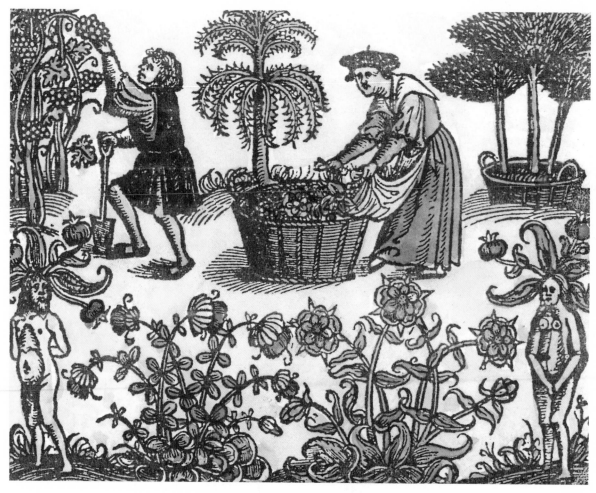

The rise of English herbalism in the 16th and 17th centuries helped to increase awareness of the healing properties of herbs.

FAMOUS HERBALISTS AND THEIR WORKS

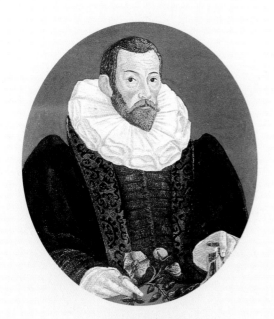

*Gardener and medical
practitioner John Gerard
cultivated plants from Europe, the
Middle East, and the Caribbean.*

JOHN GERARD 1545–1612 A gardener as well as a practitioner of medicine, he cared for several gardens during his lifetime, cultivating plant species from all over Europe, the Middle East, and even the Caribbean. His *The Herball or General Historie of Plantes* was produced in 1597, and although it was based on earlier herbals it still contains many of Gerard's personal and delightful notes regarding the growing and nurturing of plants.

JOHN PARKINSON 1567–1650 Apothecary to King James I, he produced a work entitled *Theatrum Botanicum* (*Theatre of Plants*) in 1640. In it he examined almost 4,000 plant species, many of them from exotic locations. Parkinson promoted the simplicity of herbal medicine at a time when poisonous metals and dangerously invasive techniques were being used by physicians.

NICHOLAS CULPEPER 1616–1654 Although he lived to be only 38, Culpeper's work was hugely influential with some 100 editions of his *The English Physician Enlarged* or *Complete Herbal* published in the UK and the USA since the original in 1653. Culpeper was noted for being the "peoples physician"; he treated his patients for very little money, which alienated him from other established practitioners of the time. He also insisted on using English names for plants and English remedies, and was not at all in favor of exotic ingredients. He used astrology to determine the actions of plants, regarding every plant as having an astrological ruler. Every part of the body was also governed in this way, and Culpeper generally selected plant remedies that were astrologically opposite to the body area affected by illness.

JOHN EVELYN 1620–1706 John Evelyn was a landscape gardener who was very familiar with the Chelsea Physic Garden. He wrote *A Discourse of Sallets* in 1699, encouraging people to eat more herbs in their diet. Again, he was very concerned by the strange and often poisonous remedies being used by physicians, including toxic metals, which were often being supplied at huge cost.

*Nicholas Culpeper strove to bring the
healing power of herbs within everyone's
reach, and his herbal can still be found
on modern bookshelves today.*

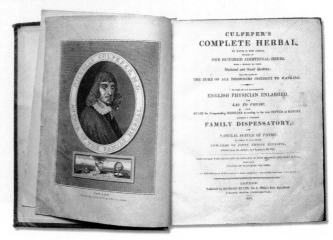

Herbs in **modern times**

Today there is a huge revival of interest in herbs in the West, not just as flavorings but also as remedies. Herbal medicine is one of the top five complementary therapies on offer in the West, with herbs being prescribed by qualified therapists to treat specific conditions in the body. Also, through the rising interest in gardening in all its forms, people are beginning to value the useful plants in their own spaces and want to learn more about them for general use.

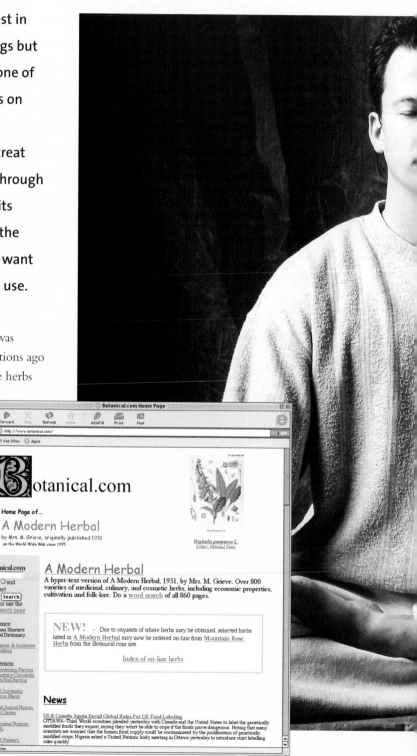

Perhaps this is simply a return to what was common knowledge just a few generations ago in our grandparents' time—how to use herbs simply and effectively to enhance food and maintain health. For a flavor of this period, it is fascinating to consult *A Modern Herbal* by Mrs M Grieve, published in 1931 and now available on-line (www.botanical.com). Mrs. Grieve cataloged hundreds of species with precise botanical descriptions, amazing snippets of folklore, and recipes, many of which must have predated the Industrial Revolution in Britain when the largely land-based population moved to the cities. Her work shows that a great deal of herbal knowledge did survive, despite medical changes.

Ayurveda is an Indian holistic healing system. It combines yoga postures, breathing exercises, and purification techniques with the healing power of herbs.

Female healers in Peru, who are known as curanderas, use a range of traditional herbal remedies such as infusions in their work.

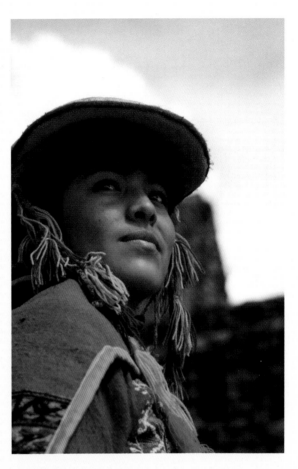

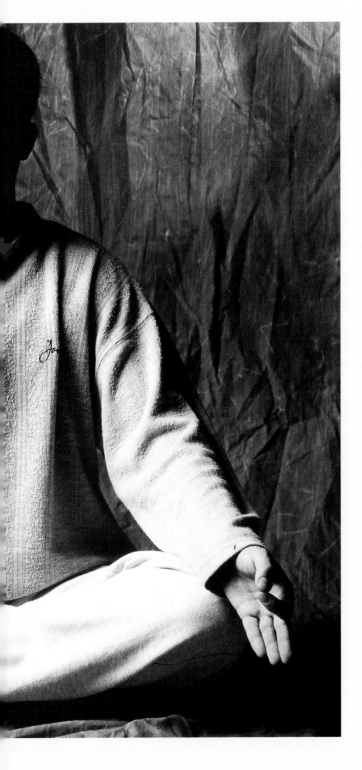

During the 18th and 19th centuries, herbal medicine fell out of use in the West as recourse to synthetic drugs increased, though the well-established herbal traditions of India, China, and the East continued as before. Toward the end of the second millennium, the return to natural remedies in the West coincided with a rising interest in the traditional medicines of the East, including Traditional Chinese Medicine or Ayurvedic principles, which emphasize the maintenance of health as well as the treatment of disease.

Today, in countries such as Korea and Cuba, herbal medicine is officially approved and available as an alternative to conventional drug therapy—the patient has that choice. In the Amazon rainforest, Kayapo medicine men are still discovering and using plants for healing. In Peru, *curanderas* (female healers) prescribe their infusions and remedies. Herbs are everywhere, and every culture still has its traditional remedies.

Herbs in your **environment**

Many of us have gardens filled with flowers of every shape and color, or balconies with pots, or maybe even just a sunny window sill on which to grow plants. Why grow herbs in particular? Perhaps because just living alongside them has subtle and wonderful effects on the senses. They are uplifting and will look attractive in any place in the home.

TO SOOTHE THE EYES

The sight of a warm brick wall where sun-loving rosemary, Greek oregano, melissa, and summer savory nestle in beds below an apricot tree trained on to a trellis, or a pergola covered in the gorgeous ample pink blooms of *Rosa Centifolia* close to a seat covered in Roman camomile, or a gray-green delicately merged bed of santolina blended with helichrysum— all these combine their colors beautifully. No garish shades here: these are the subtly lovely flowers and leaves of the herbs, whose presence is gentle and restful to the eye. Medieval herb gardens in castles were designed to provide arbors, leafy hideaways that were beautiful to look upon and enjoy.

HEAVENLY SCENTS

Herbs release wonderful fragrances into the air when the leaves or flowers are rubbed between the fingers. The eucalyptus and citrusy notes of myrtle leaves; the soft, sweet, and slightly fresh aroma of lavender; the green herbal notes of tarragon; the summer-sweet softness of elderflowers, the rich fresh pungency of sage or the clovelike tang of basil—all captivate the sense of smell. It is such a simple reaction to stop and really inhale a wonderful aroma, closing the eyes and letting the fragrance soothe you. Many wonderful gardens for blind or other sensorily impaired people make great use of scented herbs and flowers.

REST AND WELL-BEING

Your herb garden, balcony, or sunny windowsill can easily help you find a haven of tranquility and peace away from the bustle of the world. Particularly on summer evenings, after the day's work, to sit among the herbs and inhale the fragrances released by the warm weather is a wonderful and simple way to find tranquility. It is a balm to the soul just to sit and be. In the 7th century CE, Chinese sage Wang Wei said:

Look to the perfumes of leaves and flowers
for peace of mind and joy of life.

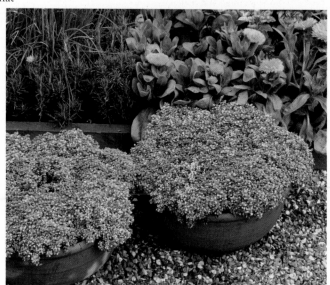

Potted herbs placed in strategic positions can soften borders and straight paths. They are also very convenient because they can be lifted and placed in different spots.

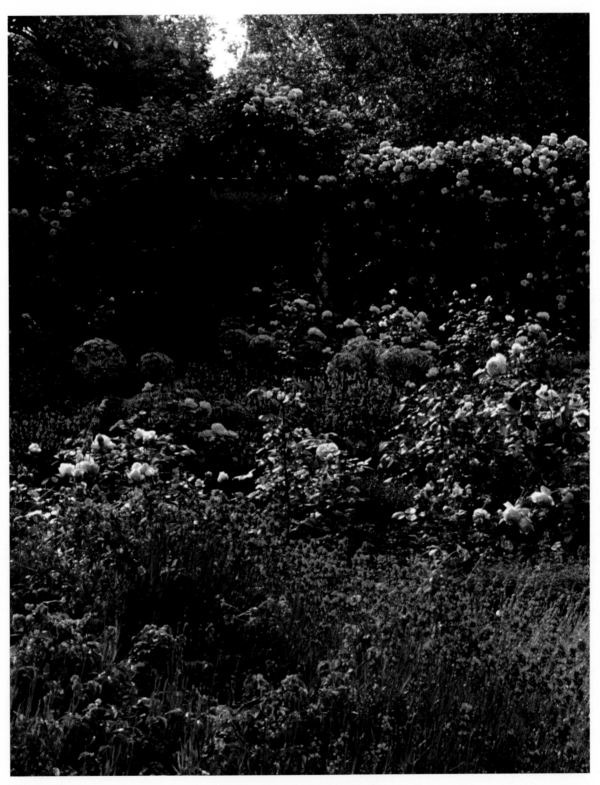

*Flowering herbs such as lavender can add a
riot of color to any garden and delight the
senses with wafts of enticing fragrances.*

Growing herbs

"MARY, MARY, QUITE CONTRARY, HOW DOES YOUR GARDEN GROW?"
The first line from the old nursery rhyme asks a useful question. If you are going to plan a herb garden, it is important to think about why you want to grow the plants and how you will use them. Growing your own medicinal herbs will boost your health, knowledge, and confidence.

A MEDICINAL GARDEN

If you want to plant herbs for medicinal use, you will need a sunny and well-sheltered area because many medicinal herbs need warmth to produce their active ingredients. In medieval monasteries, the herb garden was often walled to provide shelter and protection for the precious plants that were used to make remedies. Easy access to the plants is important; if your vital herb is difficult to reach, then you will not use it. Considering the height and likely spread of a plant is also necessary; most garden centers provide this information on plant labels. You should also bear in mind that herbs such as mint tend to take over and overrun a garden, so they are best planted in pots.

It is important to plan your garden to get the most out of the space available: pay particular attention to sunny and shady spots, and any sheltered areas.

MEDICINAL HERBS
ANGELICA, CALENDULA, COMFREY, FEVERFEW, LOVAGE, ST JOHN'S WORT, VALERIAN

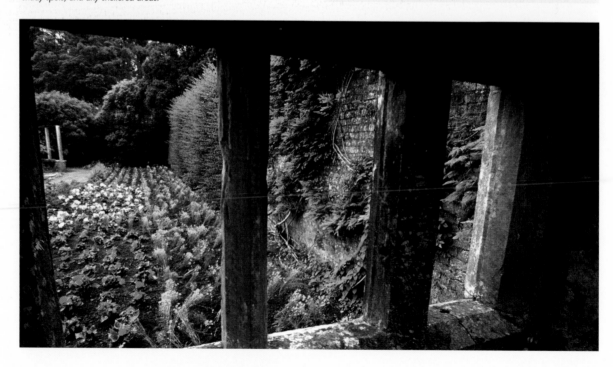

A kitchen garden needs to be as close to your home as possible, preferably near to the kitchen door, to ensure easy access to your herbs.

AN ORNAMENTAL GARDEN

If you want to create a lovely garden to please the senses with color and fragrance, you may like the idea of the more formal knot garden, where a border of box hedge encloses a regular geometric shape divided into sections, each of which contains a particular herb. Often surrounded by gravel paths and given a centerpiece such as a bay tree clipped into a definite shape, this type of garden was very popular in the 16th and 17th centuries.

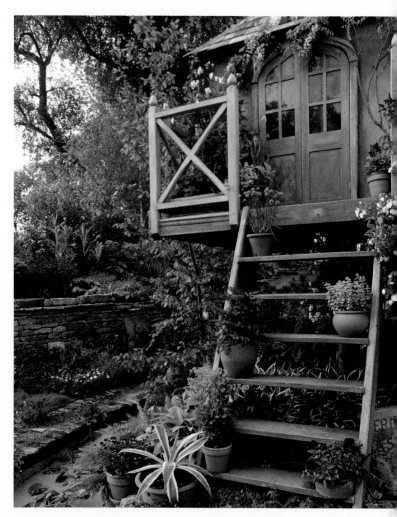

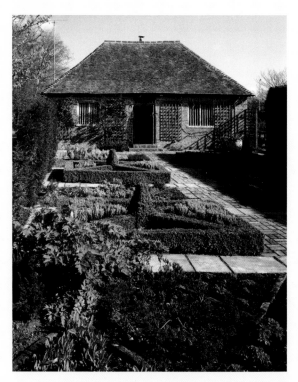

In a formal ornamental garden you can include pleasing borders of box hedge to enclose some of your herbs.

A KITCHEN GARDEN

This needs to be situated close to the house, preferably near to the door leading to the kitchen. If it is at the bottom of the garden, the herbs will not be frequently used. If you have a patio just outside your door, this may be a very good spot for several containers, which you can visit regularly to crop your herbs. Bear in mind that many of the popular kitchen herbs or spices are Mediterranean or Eastern in origin and need as much sun and warmth as possible.

ORNAMENTAL HERBS

BAY, HELICHRYSUM, LAVENDER, SAGE, SANTOLINA, SAVORY

KITCHEN HERBS

BASIL, CHERVIL, CORIANDER, FENNEL, GARLIC, MARJORAM, OREGANO, ROSEMARY, MINT

Sunny spaces and shady places

As you plan your garden, you also need to take into account how the sun travels across your space. This will show where the warmest and coolest places are, which in turn will influence the kinds of plants you decide to include.

Plant basil in a sunny place and it will flourish. It has a very pleasing fragrance and comes in different varieties, including purple basil.

BASIL

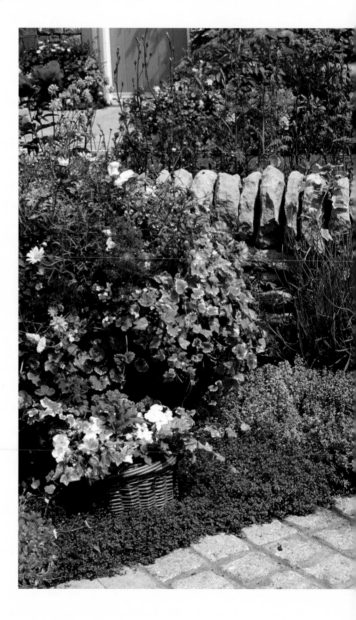

Opposite is a diagram of a typical, suburban, oblong garden that belongs to the author, showing planting areas, and the areas which are very sunny, partly shady, and fully shady. Making a sketch like this is very useful, and if it is drawn to scale it will help you set out your garden design. You can use colors to show the different light and temperature zones. If you prefer, you can simply observe where the sunny or shady spots are, but you will find it is helpful and fun to sketch your space. Some herbs prefer sun, some shade.

HERBS FOR SUN

LAVENDER, OREGANO, MARJORAM, ROSEMARY, SAGE, SAVORY, THYME, BASIL

HERBS FOR PART SHADE

CHERVIL, LADY'S MANTLE, ST JOHN'S WORT, MELISSA, PEPPERMINT, PARSLEY, SORREL

HERBS FOR TOTAL SHADE

VALERIAN, MINT, ANGELICA, LOVAGE

The majority of herbs do require some sun. Many of them also need well-drained soil, so if your soil is heavy with clay you may well need to break it up and work in some sand to help drainage. Many culinary herbs grow wild on dry, chalky, Mediterranean hillsides, so they will do well even if your garden has quite poor soil. These herbs do not require much water either, and in fact are more aromatic if they are left to grow in dry warm conditions. Sun-warmed south-facing walls retain heat and are an excellent place to grow these plants. The kinds of herbs that do tolerate some shade, such as lovage or angelica, are often found wild in woodland, growing under trees or shrubs where the soil is more moist. They will often have lush green leaves due to the high levels of nutrients available to them.

By planting in line with the microclimate zones in your garden, you are duplicating the original growing conditions of the plants you choose, and your plants will respond by growing successfully for you.

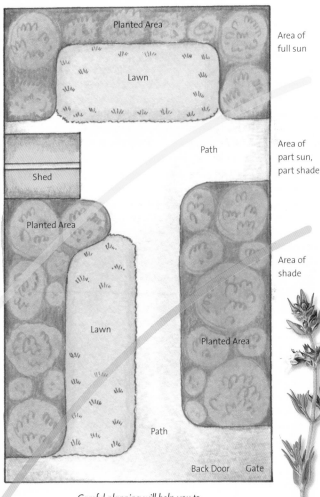

Careful planning will help you to make the most of the light and shade in your garden.

Plant herbs that like the hot sun near sun-warmed south-facing walls, and plants that can tolerate shade, such as lovage or angelica, under trees or shrubs.

THYME

Beautiful by design

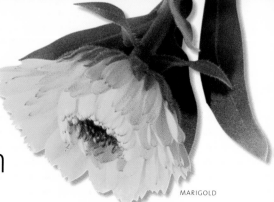

MARIGOLD

You can plant herbs in zones in your existing garden as we have just seen, but what about creating a totally new space for your herbs? Here are three ideas with accompanying sketches.

A SIMPLE KNOT GARDEN

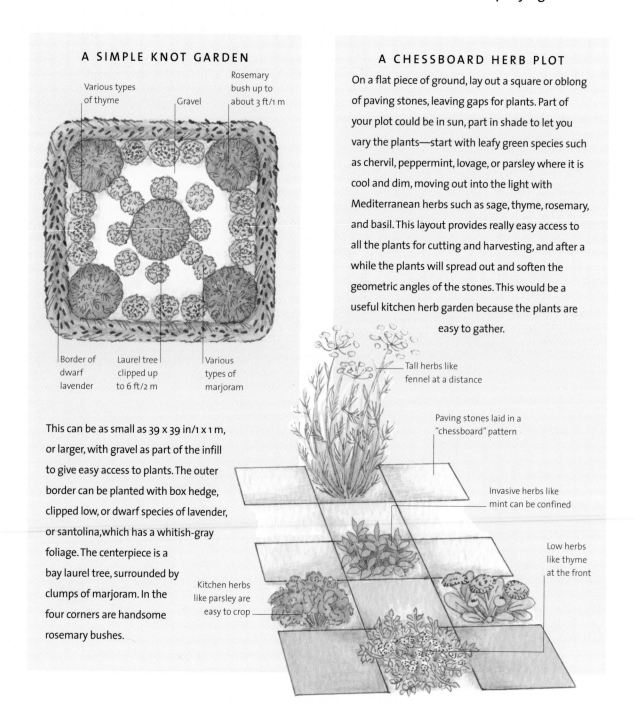

Various types of thyme

Gravel

Rosemary bush up to about 3 ft/1 m

Border of dwarf lavender

Laurel tree clipped up to 6 ft/2 m

Various types of marjoram

This can be as small as 39 x 39 in/1 x 1 m, or larger, with gravel as part of the infill to give easy access to plants. The outer border can be planted with box hedge, clipped low, or dwarf species of lavender, or santolina, which has a whitish-gray foliage. The centerpiece is a bay laurel tree, surrounded by clumps of marjoram. In the four corners are handsome rosemary bushes.

A CHESSBOARD HERB PLOT

On a flat piece of ground, lay out a square or oblong of paving stones, leaving gaps for plants. Part of your plot could be in sun, part in shade to let you vary the plants—start with leafy green species such as chervil, peppermint, lovage, or parsley where it is cool and dim, moving out into the light with Mediterranean herbs such as sage, thyme, rosemary, and basil. This layout provides really easy access to all the plants for cutting and harvesting, and after a while the plants will spread out and soften the geometric angles of the stones. This would be a useful kitchen herb garden because the plants are easy to gather.

Tall herbs like fennel at a distance

Paving stones laid in a "chessboard" pattern

Invasive herbs like mint can be confined

Low herbs like thyme at the front

Kitchen herbs like parsley are easy to crop

A MEDIEVAL GARDEN

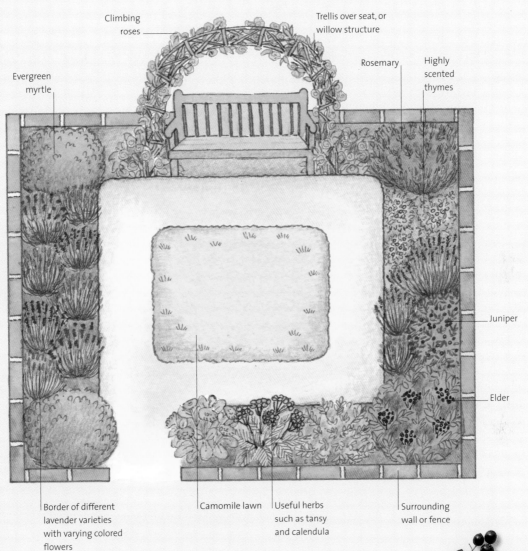

Climbing roses

Trellis over seat, or willow structure

Rosemary

Highly scented thymes

Evergreen myrtle

Juniper

Elder

Border of different lavender varieties with varying colored flowers

Camomile lawn

Useful herbs such as tansy and calendula

Surrounding wall or fence

This takes more space and planning, and includes a surrounding wall or trellis with a seat, around which are so-called "old" roses, such as *Rosa gallica*, Apothecary's rose. Climbing roses could be trained over the top of seat. In the center is a camomile lawn, and the beds are planted with all manner of old strewing herbs like lavender and rosemary, and medicinal herbs like feverfew, lady's mantle, and melissa. Evergreen bushes of myrtle and juniper add contrast. This would be a truly healing garden, a balm to the senses.

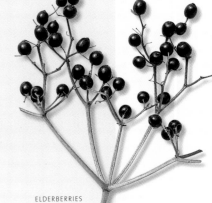

ELDERBERRIES

SAND

Miniature **herb** Garden

Patios, yards, and balconies can be transformed by planting aromatic and useful herbs in a whole variety of pots or containers and arranging them in a pleasing display. The resulting plants can still provide a useful crop for kitchen and medicinal use.

TYPES OF POTS

Herbs do well in terracotta or ceramic pots, but be aware that these are very heavy and may be difficult to move if you want to overwinter your herbs in a greenhouse or indoors! A whole range of troughs, barrels, even old chimney pots can make a varied display. Strawberry pots with several openings let a variety of herbs be planted very compactly if space is lacking.

Avoid over-rich soils when potting your herbs —when in doubt, ask at your local garden center.

PLANTING

Pots need good drainage; a layer of broken crockery or gravel needs to go in first to let water drain through. Blend one-third standard potting compost, one-third garden soil, and one-third coarse sand to make a basic planting mixture. Do not give herbs over-rich soil because they will not thrive. If you are using a strawberry pot, then plant from the bottom upward as you gradually fill the pot with soil. If you are using a trough or a large pot, bear in mind that the herbs will spread out, so leave plenty of space between plants or use one pot for a single plant. Containers are very good for planting invasive plants like mint or melissa.

Pots come in a wide range of materials, colors, and finishes, and can transform any patio, terrace, yard, or balcony.

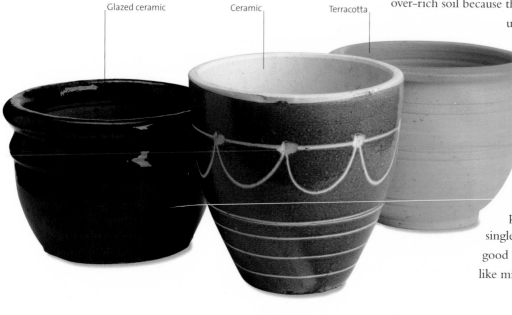

Glazed ceramic   Ceramic   Terracotta

WATERING

Your container herbs
will need watering, but
be careful not to overdo it.
Keep the soil moist but never
waterlogged. It is best to water in
the mornings or evenings on hot
days. If you have been away and
forgotten your pots, then the best thing to
do is to stand them in a container of water
for about 10 minutes so the water is soaked
up through the roots.

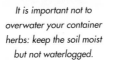

*It is important not to
overwater your container
herbs: keep the soil moist
but not waterlogged.*

FEEDING

Commercial plant feeds are not really suitable for
herbs and should be used only in moderation. You
can make your own plant food instead by filling a
bucket full of either nettle or comfrey leaves, then
covering them with water and leaving it to stand in
the sun for a few weeks. Dilute one part of the brew
with 10 parts water and feed the herbs once in spring
and again in midsummer.

OBTAINING HERBS TO GROW

Good garden centers and herb
nurseries are excellent sources of
plants to start your herb garden. You
may also be lucky enough to have
friends who may give you cuttings of
their plants to grow, and as your plants
become established you can increase your
own supply by the following methods:

TAKING CUTTINGS

Use this method for aromatic woody
shrubs like lavender, sage, rosemary. In
late spring/early summer, select a non-flowering stem
and pull or cut gently from the parent plant, leaving a
little "heel" of bark at the base. Press into compost
around the edge of a plant pot.

DIVISION OF ROOTS

Use this method for mint, camomile, lovage, angelica.
In late spring or early fall, dig up the whole
plant and gently prize apart the roots or
divide with a knife and replant the clumps
separately.

SOW SEEDS

Collect seed from the previous year
and plant up in early spring,
transplanting seedlings out to the
garden or pot later in the season.

*You can find a wide range of herbs from
your local garden center or herb nursery.
If you are planting herbs from seed, make
sure you label the pots.*

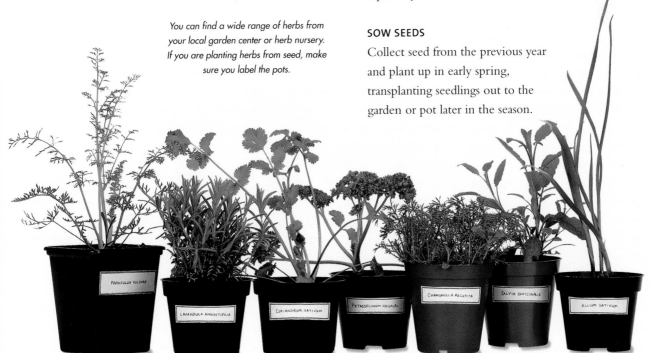

HARVESTING AND PRESERVING YOUR HERBS

Having planted and produced your herbs, you may wish to pick them and use them. Alternatively, you may wish to prepare them for storage through the winter. This is a very satisfying task as you visit each plant you have grown, and observe how it has changed through the growing season.

Many herbs, such as marjoram or rosemary, are available from spring to fall, and others require harvesting at specific times.

PICKING

Leaves of aromatic herbs like basil, thyme, peppermint, or melissa need to be picked for drying just before the plant flowers. Cropping is best done in a sunny morning after dew has dried. If you want to pick the whole flowering top, such as St John's wort, you need to collect it as the flowers are opening. Seeds should be collected just before they fall to the ground; cut the whole flowering top and suspend it upside down in a paper bag to catch the seeds.

SEASONAL HARVESTING

LATE SPRING: stems of angelica, borage leaves, fennel leaves, feverfew leaves, rosemary leaves, sorrel leaves

EARLY SUMMER: basil leaves, elder flowers, melissa leaves, lovage leaves, parsley leaves, calendula flowers, sage leaves

MIDSUMMER: angelica seed, camomile flowers, lavender flowers, marjoram leaves, mint leaves, St John's wort flowering top, summer savory leaves, yarrow flowering top

LATE SUMMER: chervil leaves, coriander seeds, elderberries, fennel seed, juniper berries, lovage seed, garlic bulbs

EARLY FALL: angelica root, dandelion root

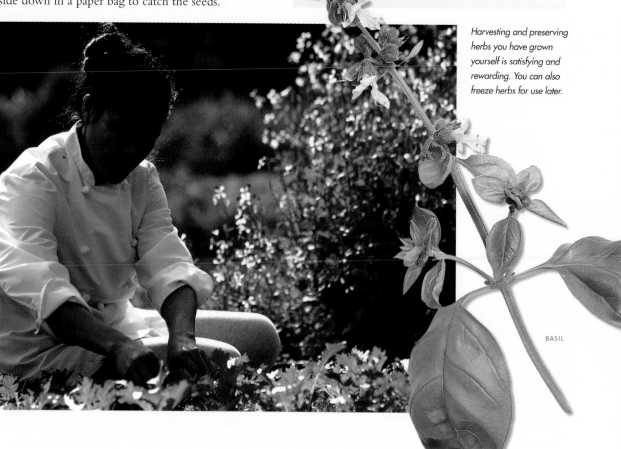

Harvesting and preserving herbs you have grown yourself is satisfying and rewarding. You can also freeze herbs for use later.

BASIL

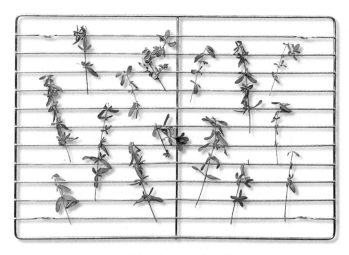

Try drying delicate flower heads and leaves by placing them on a cooking rack; this will help prevent breaking as they dry.

PRESERVING HERBS

Drying Tie herbs into bunches with about 10 stems each. Delicate flowering tops or flowers should be laid to dry on a wire rack (such as that used for letting food cool), or spread with brown paper with holes cut in it. Hang bunches or place trays in a well-ventilated attic, dry shady room, or in an airing cupboard with the door left open. The temperature should not exceed 90°F (33°C). The herbs are ready when they are brittle and break easily. Store in airtight jars.

Freezing A few sprigs of herbs at a time can be placed in small plastic bags and then frozen. Pinches of leaves can be placed in an ice-making tray and topped up with water, then frozen. Try freezing peppermint or borage leaves this way and add them straight into summer wine punches.

You can put sprigs of fresh herbs in small plastic bags and then freeze them throughout the winter for a ready supply.

DRYING HERBS

DRYING LEAVES, STEMS, AND AERIAL PARTS

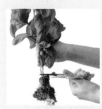

1 First harvest them by cutting with a sharp knife or secateurs to prevent tearing.

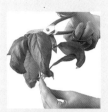

2 Strip the leaves or flowers from the main stem. For some herbs you can dry the stems too.

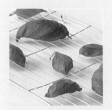

3 Spread out separately on a drying rack and leave to dry in the sun or a warm place until they are brittle and crumble easily.

DRYING ROOTS

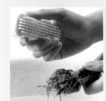

1 First unearth them gently. Wash the root to remove all remaining dirt. Scrub with a nail brush if necessary.

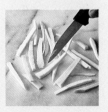

2 Strip the leaves or flowers from the main stem. For some herbs you can dry the stems too.

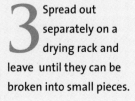

3 Spread out separately on a drying rack and leave until they can be broken into small pieces.

Herbs in the **wild**

Herbs were, of course, originally wild plants, and in many of their native habitats they still grow and multiply as they have always done. In Provence in Southern France, you may see glorious lavender bushes growing straight out of rocks. On wasteland, you may find yarrow or elder trees growing with lush abundance. These days, in the interests of preserving native species, environmental concerns are important when it comes to picking wild plants.

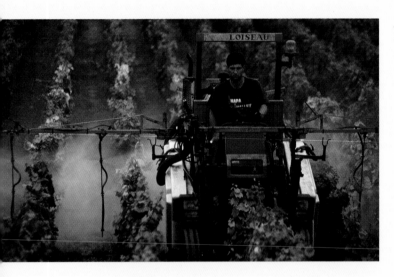

Modern agricultural methods can cause widespread damage to wild plants and contaminate them with chemicals and toxins.

LOCATION

It is very important to respect wild species growing in woodland, wetlands, or areas of natural beauty. It can be very rewarding to study, draw, or photograph plants in their true habitat to learn more about how they grow and what conditions suit them; however, the local environment should be disturbed as little as possible. There may be local by-laws prohibiting picking, which need to be observed.

RARITY

Many wild species are threatened with extinction as the ecosystems where they would naturally thrive are threatened by industrial or urban spread. As far as possible, habitats where rare plants grow should be protected and left alone.

POLLUTION

Modern agricultural methods and industrial wastes are responsible for widespread environmental damage. Wild plants that manage to survive despite this may be contaminated with chemical residues, or if they grow near roadsides they may contain toxins.

IDENTIFICATION

Many wild species look similar to domesticated varieties of similar plants but may, in fact, be poisonous. Use a plant guide with photographs rather than line drawings, and if in doubt do not pick at all. If you are confident in your identification, pick only from a plentiful supply of the plant, leaving a good amount behind for it to restore itself.

Our ancestors were quite used to picking wild herbs to supplement what they grew themselves; common land, woodland, or wasteland were often visited in this way. In the 17th century, Culpeper mentioned Lincoln's Inn Fields in London, England as an open area where people could find plants. It is a sobering fact that many of our wild spaces are rapidly disappearing; all the more reason to treat what remains as precious to ourselves and our children.

A–Z of **herbs**

The next section contains profiles of 40 common herbs with botanical information, historical references, tips for cultivation, and uses in the kitchen and for general health maintenance. It is not a good idea to take the same herb medicinally for more than a few days without professional guidance. When they are used in moderation, herbs can help the body to restore itself very gently and effectively, but if you are unwell, pregnant, have a recognized medical problem, or are taking medication, consult your doctor or a qualified medical herbalist before using herbs on yourself. Herbs are powerful natural substances and should be used with care and respect.

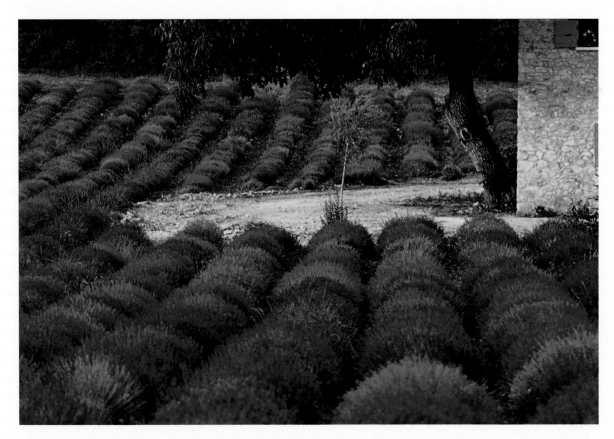

Yarrow

Achillea millefolium (Compositae)

DATA FILE

PLANT DESCRIPTION: Perennial herb with creeping roots and erect, furrowed, downy stems (up to 2 ft/60 cm), feathery leaves, and flat heads of small whitish flowers from midsummer to fall. The whole plant is very fragrant.

CULTIVATION: Grows wild in meadows and fields; if cultivated, it will spread, so it may need containment. Existing plants can be divided or seed sown in spring. It prefers full sun and well-drained soil.

PLANT PARTS USED: Leaves and flowering tops (picked before fully in bloom, dried outdoors in the shade). Flowering tops also yield an essential oil.

MAIN USES: Yarrow blended with elderflower and peppermint is an excellent infusion for colds and flu. It has a blood-purifying effect and encourages sweating. A cool infusion, poultice, or ointment of yarrow can be used on wounds.

CAUTION
Use with care on sensitive skin and only for short periods of time.

YARROW

HISTORY

Yarrow has enjoyed other names such as "Staunchweed" or "Soldiers' woundwort," which link to its wound-healing properties. In Roman times, it was known as *herba militaris*, the military herb. The name *Achillea* refers to Achilles, one of the heroes of the Trojan War.

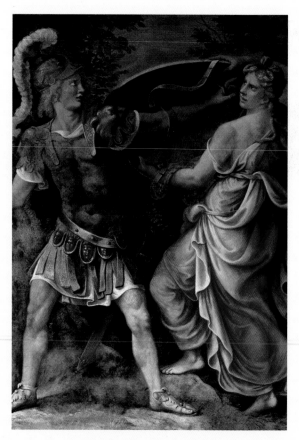

Achilles, one of the heroes of the Trojan war, was reputed to have used yarrow to heal battle wounds.

Chervil
Anthriscus cerefolium (Umbelliferae)

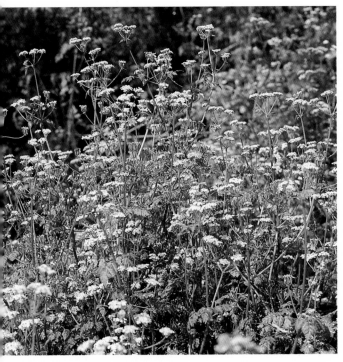

ABOVE *This annual herb has finely grooved stems and small white flowers. It grows freely on wasteland and is cultivated all over the world.*

BELOW *Fresh chervil leaves make an excellent garnish for soups and salads. The herb is excellent for supporting the digestive system.*

DATA FILE

PLANT DESCRIPTION: delicate annual plant (up to 2 ft/60 cm) with tapering roots, feathery foliage rather like parsley, branching stems, and flat flower heads covered in tiny white blooms.

CULTIVATION: Sow seeds in spring in well-moistened soil in full sun. It will self-seed.

USEFUL PLANT PARTS: Leaves (gathered fresh and gently dried) and roots (dug up fresh and boiled).

MAIN USES: An infusion of the leaves and stalks is useful for indigestion. The roots eaten as a vegetable are said to have a soothing effect on the stomach. The fresh leaves are used as a flavoring in soups, salads, and garnishes.

CAUTION
It is important to plant the correct botanical species (above). Some species of wild chervil are poisonous.

HISTORY

Traditionally, several plants with the common name "chervil" were used. Culpeper employed it medicinally as a digestive and respiratory tonic. Gerard comments, "The leaves of sweet Chervill are exceeding good, wholesome, and pleasant among other sallad herbs." It has always been popular in France as a culinary flavoring.

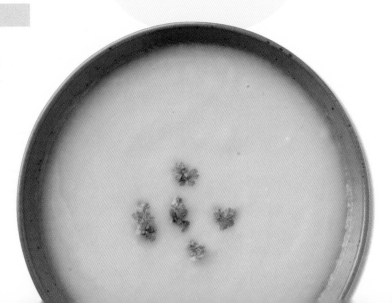

Tarragon
Artemisia dracunculus (Compositae)

DATA FILE

PLANT DESCRIPTION: Perennial herb, shrubby and dense (up to 3 ft/1 m) with narrow, pointed, smooth, dark green leaves and spikes of small, whitish-yellow flowers. Highly aromatic, it spreads easily due to invasive roots.

CULTIVATION: Tarragon is usually propagated by division of roots in March and April, or by cuttings. This herb needs warmth and sun and a dry situation, well-drained soil, and protection from frost. It also needs to be cut right back before the winter.

PLANT PARTS USED: Leaves (fresh or dried in shade to preserve aroma).

MAIN USES: Infusion of the leaves helps toothache, indigestion, and insomnia and acts as a general tonic. Tarragon is a key flavoring in French cooking, used in salads, sauces, herb seasonings, flavored vinegars, and chicken dishes.

Tarragon is a popular flavoring in French cuisine. It helps to sweeten the breath and improves the digestive process.

CAUTION
Avoid exposure to sunlight after treating skin—this plant can cause photosensitivity.

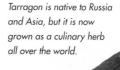

Tarragon is native to Russia and Asia, but it is now grown as a culinary herb all over the world.

HISTORY

The plant is found growing from China and Mongolia through Europe to North America. The name "tarragon" derives from French *estragon*, which in turn comes from the Latin *dracunculus* meaning "little dragon." It was famed as a cure for the poison of insect or snakebites.

Oat

Avena sativa (Graminea)

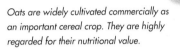

Oats are widely cultivated commercially as an important cereal crop. They are highly regarded for their nutritional value.

DATA FILE

PLANT DESCRIPTION: Annual grown as an important cereal crop. Tall stems (up to 3 ft/1 m) with a sheath of long, narrow leaves. The drooping flower heads become the small, hard oat grains.

CULTIVATION: Widely grown on a commercial scale and available as various grades of whole oats, oatflakes, and oatmeal (which are best purchased from organic sources).

PLANT PARTS USED: Grains (used as food and also used medicinally).

MAIN USES: Tincture of oat may be taken for overwrought nerves, insomnia, stress, or convalescence (10–30 drops in water). Oat porridge or savory oat soup is extremely easy to digest and helps build strength after illness. Infusion of oats helps anxiety, mental fatigue, or insomnia and may be gargled to ease sore throats. Putting oatmeal in a cheesecloth bag with other herbs can be used to soften bath water and cleanse the skin.

HISTORY

Originally native to Eastern Europe, oats have been widely cultivated for thousands of years. Infused or cooked oats were often used to clarify the skin. In medieval times, the German prophetess and healer Hildegard of Bingen regarded oats as a useful nerve tonic and gastric remedy.

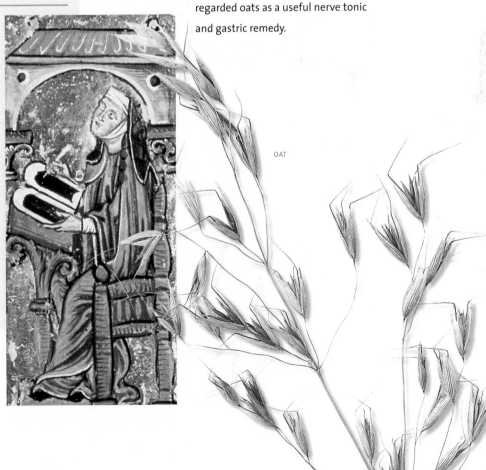

Medieval German abbess Hildegard of Bingen prized oats for their value as a nerve tonic and gastric remedy.

OAT

Borage

Borago officinalis (Boraginaceae)

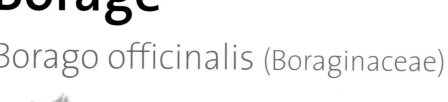

BORAGE
FLOWER

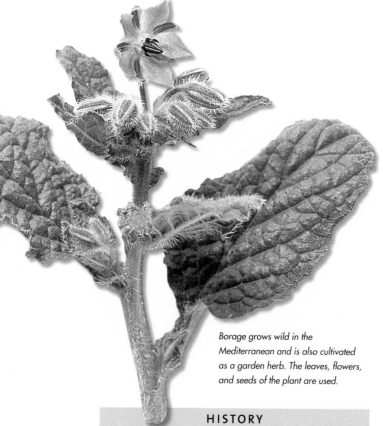

Borage grows wild in the Mediterranean and is also cultivated as a garden herb. The leaves, flowers, and seeds of the plant are used.

HISTORY

Traditionally used as a restorative herb, the leaves have a cucumber-like fragrance and were used to make refreshing summer drinks. Gerard maintained, "It maketh a man merrie and joyfull."

DATA FILE

PLANT DESCRIPTION: Vigorous annual herb with hollow bristly stems (up to 3 ft/90 cm), broad, oval, hairy leaves, clusters of blue, star-shaped flowers, followed by oval seed clusters. Very attractive to bees, it spreads easily and often grows wild on waste ground.

CULTIVATION: Flourishes in ordinary soil and can be propagated by division of root clumps, but left alone it will seed itself yearly. It grows best in full sun.

USEFUL PLANT PARTS: Leaves (used fresh), flowers (picked fresh), and seeds (dried).

MAIN USES: Borage is used to help colds, flu, or bronchitis by promoting sweating; an infusion of the leaves is taken twice daily. Commercially grown borage produces a seed oil rich in GLA (gamma-linoleic acid, which is also found in evening primrose). Borage oil capsules may improve dry skin, menstrual imbalances, and even rheumatoid arthritis. Borage flowers can be eaten in salads or used decoratively on cakes.

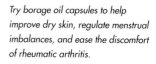

Try borage oil capsules to help improve dry skin, regulate menstrual imbalances, and ease the discomfort of rheumatic arthritis.

Calendula (marigold)

Calendula officinalis (Compositae)

MAKING A TINCTURE

8–10½ oz/220–310 g of leaves
1 cup/250 ml 80% vodka and
scant 3 cups/750 ml water

*Place leaves into a blender and pour in
the alcohol. When blended, pour into
a dark glass jar and cover with an
airtight lid. Shake well and label.
Store for two days in a cool dark
place, giving it a shake once a day.
After two days add water to the
mixture. Now leave the jar for four
weeks, in a cool, dark place,
shaking it daily.*

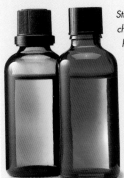

*Strain the tincture through a
cheesecloth bag overnight until you
have all the liquid. A wine press
would give the best result.*

*Pour into sterilized dark bottles,
then label and store in a dark,
cool place. The tincture can be
decanted into 2 fl oz (50 ml)
tincture bottles for personal use.*

DATA FILE

PLANT DESCRIPTION: Herb normally planted as an annual, with slightly sticky stems (up to 2 ft/60 cm), long, hairy leaves and yellow-orange flowers from early summer. This is the only species of marigold to have any medicinal value.

CULTIVATION: Sow seeds in full sun or part shade, thinning out seedlings to leave room for the plant to spread. Deadheading prolongs the flowering season. Calendula self-seeds itself easily.

USEFUL PLANT PARTS: Leaves and flowers (need quick drying in the dark, spread on sheets of paper).

MAIN USES: The flowers applied either as a cold infusion or as an ointment relieve swelling and soothe dry, sore skin. A hot infusion of the flowers drunk twice a day can help indigestion and stomach cramps. The young leaves can be eaten in salads.

TIP

if you prefer to
use 37–45% proof
vodka, do not add
the water
mixture

HISTORY

Well-known to old herbalists as a garden flower for use in cookery and medicine. Shakespeare mentions the "Marigold that goes to bed wi'th'sun, and with him rises weeping," alluding to the flowers closing up at sunset. Marigolds were thought to strengthen the eyesight and were also sometimes used to make a yellow dye.

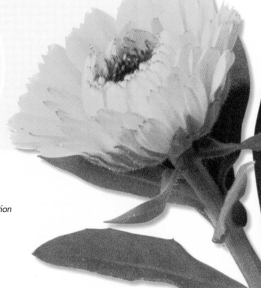

*Marigold is a popular garden
plant. It is very helpful for skin
problems and soothes indigestion
and stomach cramps.*

CORIANDER
SEEDS

Coriander (Cilantro)

Coriandrum sativum (Umbelliferae)

DATA FILE

PLANT DESCRIPTION: Strong-smelling plant with slender stems (up to 2 ft/60 cm), rich, green, fernlike leaves, and flat flower heads of pinkish-white flowers in midsummer, followed by reddish-brown seed capsules.

CULTIVATION: Seeds can be sown in April, requiring a well-drained soil with a little lime, full sun, and protection from wind. Pinching out the flower heads encourages bushier leaf production. It makes a useful container herb.

USEFUL PLANT PARTS: Leaves (fresh) and seeds (dried—the longer the seeds are left, the better the aroma).

MAIN USES: The fresh leaves add a piquant taste to salads, soups, and Indian dishes; the ground seeds act as a digestive stimulant by increasing gastric juices and are used to flavor curries.

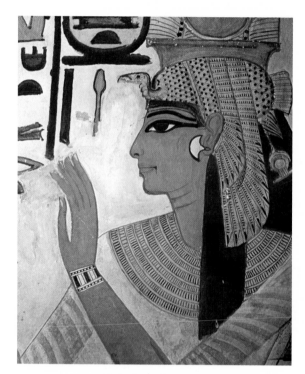

Coriander seeds were very popular in ancient Egypt, and were mentioned in the Ebers papyrus, which dates from around 1500 BCE.

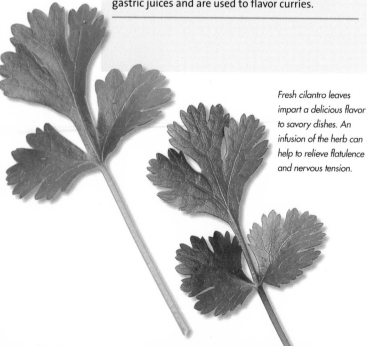

Fresh cilantro leaves impart a delicious flavor to savory dishes. An infusion of the herb can help to relieve flatulence and nervous tension.

HISTORY

The seeds are one of the oldest recorded spices, mentioned in ancient Egyptian documents from over 1,000 years ago. It was brought to Britain by the Romans; it is still commonly used in Middle Eastern, South American, and Indian cooking. In ancient Greek times, the seeds and herb were employed as digestive tonics.

Ground carrot seeds taken as an infusion are very helpful for easing colic and stomach cramps.

Carrot
Daucus carota (Umbelliferae)

DATA FILE

PLANT DESCRIPTION: Robust plant with tall branched stems (up to 2 ft/60 cm), fine, feathery leaves, flattened flower heads with many tiny pinkish-white flowers, becoming flat seeds in a spiked case; the root is orange-red and is familiar as a vegetable.

CULTIVATION: Originally a wild plant favoring seaside coasts and wayside locations, carrots grow best in sandy, well-drained soil. Seeds may be obtained from good garden suppliers. In the garden, several crops of carrots can be sown in one season from February through to August.

USEFUL PLANT PARTS: Seeds (dried), roots (eaten as a vegetable), leaves (used fresh).

MAIN USES: Carrot seeds ground into a powder and infused are helpful for colic and stomach cramps. An infusion of the leaves cleanses and detoxifies the body, helping gout and urinary stones. The roots are an excellent source of Vitamin A and soothe the digestive tract.

CAUTION
Carrot seeds can promote menstruation, so do not use seeds during pregnancy.

CARROT LEAVES

Carrots once grew wild in coastal areas, but now they are cultivated commercially and in gardens.

HISTORY

In culinary and medicinal use since very ancient times; it is mentioned by the ancient Greek herbalist Dioscorides in the 1st century CE as a digestive tonic. Carrot seeds were employed by Culpeper to help indigestion, wind, and colic, as well as gout.

CARROT FLOWER

Echinacea (Purple coneflower)

Echinacea angustifolia, Echinacea purpurea (Compositae)

DATA FILE

PLANT DESCRIPTION: An attractive plant (up to 18 in/45 cm) with rich purple flowers around a high central cone. The roots are tapering and fibrous with a faint aroma. It is originally native to the USA, now also cultivated in Britain.

CULTIVATION: May be grown from seed sown in spring, or divided roots of existing plants.

USEFUL PLANT PARTS: Roots (dried or fresh, prepared as a decoction or tincture) and flowering tops (infused, left to cool, for external use)

MAIN USES: Tincture of the root is regarded as one of the best preventive remedies for enhancing immune function, especially for chronic conditions. A cool wash made from infused flowers and leaves is helpful for itching skin or insect bites and stings.

Echinacea was a popular herbal remedy among Native Americans, including the Sioux who took it as a remedy for snake bites, and the Comanche who used it for sore throats.

HISTORY

Another name for echinacea was Kansas snakeroot, and it had a strong reputation among Native Americans and frontiersmen as a healer of snake bites, as well as a cleanser of infected wounds. Modern herbalists regard it as one of the best blood-cleansing herbs, and a powerful immune-system stimulant.

Echinacea has beautiful purple flowers and is native to the United States, although it is now grown commercially in Europe as well.

Fennel

Foeniculum vulgare (Umbelliferae)

DATA FILE

PLANT DESCRIPTION: A biennial plant with erect, blue-green, branching stems (up to 6 ft/1.8 m). The leaves are soft, dark green, and feathery; flower stalks culminate in flat heads covered with little yellow flowers, followed by tiny, egg-shaped seed pods.

CULTIVATION: Seeds that are sown in April need plenty of sun and light moist soil. Deadheading encourages bushier leaf production. The plant self-seeds easily, and old plants need removing every three to four years.

USEFUL PLANT PARTS: Leaves (fresh or dried), and seeds (dried).

MAIN USES: The leaves in a hot infusion help indigestion, wind, or colic; a cool infusion soothes tired eyes. The seeds can be chewed after meals to aid digestion. Fennel leaves are a key flavoring in southern Mediterranean soups, fish, and meat dishes.

Hot fennel tea is a soothing remedy for indigestion, wind, colic, and irritable bowel problems. It can also help to ease anxiety.

Fennel is a very versatile herb. It is very popular in cookery and medicine, and in cosmetics, including toothpastes and soaps.

HISTORY

Fennel has a history of use throughout Europe, across the Mediterranean and all the way to India. The Romans were fond of it in sweet and savory dishes. Herbalist John Parkinson (see page 13) in 1640 tells us that "the culinary use came from Italy; the taste being sweete and somewhat hot helpeth to digest the crude qualitie of fish and other meats..."

Witch hazel

Hamamelis virginiana (Hamamelidaceae)

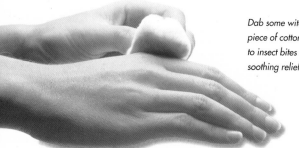

Dab some witch hazel onto a piece of cotton wool and apply it to insect bites and stings for soothing relief.

HISTORY

Originally native to the eastern US and Canada, witch hazel was a traditional remedy of Native American medicine men, who used it to treat wounds and stop bleeding.

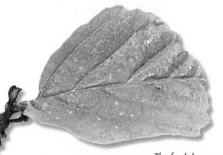

The fresh leaves and twigs, and flowering young twigs, are used to make the herbal preparations.

DATA FILE

PLANT DESCRIPTION: Deciduous perennial shrub or small tree (up to 12 ft/4 m). The soft, serrated leaves resemble hazel, and the ragged, yellow flowers bloom from the fall onward.

CULTIVATION: The witch hazel tree prefers a lime-free soil and full sun, growing well against a wall. It sends out suckers, which can be transplanted for new plants. The yellow blooms are very cheering in the wintertime.

PLANT PARTS USED: Leaves and twigs (for a tincture), flowering young twigs (for a distillation of witch hazel water).

MAIN USES: Witch hazel ointment is very soothing to varicose veins or hemorrhoids, bruises or sprains. A compress of witch hazel water is very effective at stopping bleeding. The water is also a very useful natural skincare ingredient, working well on oily or combination skins as a freshener. Witch hazel water also soothes insect bites and stings (apply on a cotton wool pad).

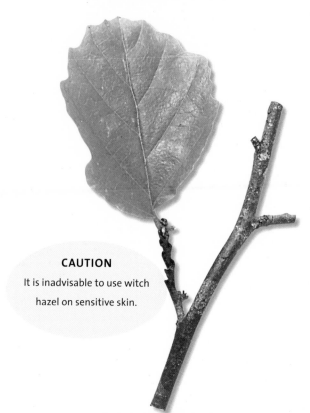

CAUTION

It is inadvisable to use witch hazel on sensitive skin.

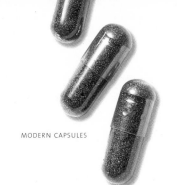

MODERN CAPSULES

St John's wort

Hypericum perforatum (Guttiferae)

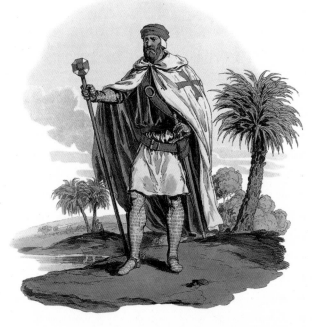

The knights of St John of Jerusalem are believed to have used St John's wort to heal battle wounds during the crusades.

BELOW *St John's wort promotes healing of wounds and burns, soothes the pain of gout and arthritis, and helps to ease depression.*

HISTORY

In crusader times, the knights of St John of Jerusalem are said to have used the herb in wound-healing, and "wort" is an old word for herb. Many superstitions are attached to this plant; traditionally, sprigs of it were hung in doorways or windows to keep away evil spirits.

DATA FILE

PLANT DESCRIPTION: A low, evergreen shrub with stout, creeping roots and erect stems (up to 3 ft/90 cm) with two parallel vertical ridges. The small, green leaves are speckled with tiny translucent glands. Golden yellow flowers occur in late summer.

CULTIVATION: Can be grown in sun or part shade; needs a good well-drained soil. Roots of existing plants can be divided in spring, when any frost-damaged stems should be pruned.

PLANT PARTS USED: Young leaves or flowers (fresh or dried in shade).

MAIN USES: Macerating the leaves and flowers in vegetable oil makes an excellent preparation for slow-healing cuts, wounds, burns, or scalds. Infusion of the leaves and flowers helps gout and arthritis. St John's wort is given in tablets or capsules to help depression or anxiety.

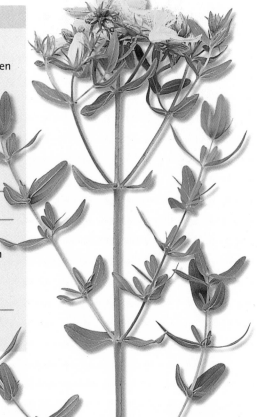

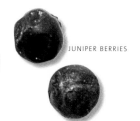

JUNIPER BERRIES

Juniper

Juniperus communis (Cupressaceae)

HISTORY

During the time of bubonic plague, juniper berries were regarded as having protective qualities. Culpeper used juniper as a diuretic and strongly tonic remedy. Juniper berries are used to make gin. In Switzerland, a jam of juniper berries is still eaten as a protective measure against winter colds and flu.

The juniper bush grows in Europe, the United States, and Canada. The ripe berries are harvested and dried in the sun.

Drink an infusion of juniper berries to soothe the symptoms of cystitis or improve digestion.

DATA FILE

PLANT DESCRIPTION: Evergreen shrub, can grow near ground level (prostrate form) or as tall as 20 ft/6 m. It has sharp needle-like leaves, yellowish flowers in early summer, followed by fleshy berries, which are green at first and take up to two years to ripen to a blue-black color.

CULTIVATION: Can be planted from cuttings taken in the fall. It requires a well-drained soil in an open position.

USEFUL PLANT PARTS: Ripe berries, gathered in the summer and dried in the sun.

MAIN USES: The berries yield an essential oil which is a powerful diuretic and muscle tonic. An infusion of the berries is helpful for cystitis, sluggish digestion, or poor appetite, and a steam inhalation of berries assists chesty coughs, colds, and bronchitis.

CAUTION
Do not use juniper in pregnancy or kidney disease.

Peppermint

Mentha x piperita
(Labiatae/Lamiaceae)

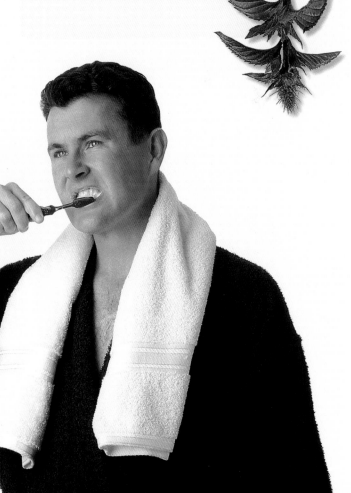

Peppermint is an invasive herb, so plant it in a container to prevent it from overrunning your garden.

DATA FILE

PLANT DESCRIPTION: A perennial herb with very invasive roots, and tall, square, branching stems (up to 3 ft/90 cm). The leaves are dark green and slightly hairy with serrated edges. The whole plant is highly aromatic, with pink flowers in the late summer. Peppermint is a cultivated cross between water mint and spearmint.

CULTIVATION: Requires a warm spot with moist, rich soil. Once established, it spreads very vigorously and may need containment, or growing in a pot.

PLANT PARTS USED: Leaves and stems (fresh or dried).

MAIN USES: Infusion of the leaves, peppermint tea, soothes and calms indigestion, wind, or colic. Infused with yarrow and elderflower, peppermint assists the immune system in the early stages of a cold or flu. The essential oil is used to flavor toothpaste and chewing gum, in pharmaceutical preparations for aching muscles, and also in confectionery.

HISTORY

Ancient Greeks and Romans used peppermint extensively as a decoration at feasts and as an ingredient in sauces. In the 18th century, the county of Surrey in England was world-famous as a producer of the herb and essential oil.

The fresh flavor of peppermint is widely used in confectionery such as chewing gum, and in cosmetic preparations such as toothpaste.

Myrtle
Myrtus communis (Myrtaceae)

Myrtle is native to the Mediterreanean area. The flowers, leaves, twigs, and berries are used to make herbal remedies.

DATA FILE

PLANT DESCRIPTION: A very aromatic, evergreen shrub (up to 10 ft/3 m) with flaking bark and reddish brown stems. Long, oval leaves are dark green, fragrant, and glossy. Soft, white flowers in late summer are followed by dark purple berries.

CULTIVATION: Requires a fertile, well-drained soil, full sun, and a well-sheltered position if being grown in northern latitudes.

PLANT PARTS USED: Leaves and twigs (fresh or dried), flowers (fully open), and berries (fresh or dried).

MAIN USES: Crushed fresh leaves can be applied to cuts and wounds. A hot infusion of the leaves helps colds, coughs, or bronchitis and acts as an all-round tonic; a cooled infusion makes a lovely skin toner and freshener. Ointment of fresh flowers nourishes the skin.

HISTORY

Myrtle communis is native to the Mediterranean region and Greek mythology often refers to it. Sacred to Aphrodite, the Goddess of Love, it was carried by brides and worn in wedding wreaths. Flowers and leaves were ingredients of "angel's water," a 16th-century skin lotion, and myrtle is still used in cosmetic formulations today.

In ancient Greece, myrtle was considered to be sacred to Aphrodite, the Goddess of Love.

Basil (sweet)

Ocimum basilicum (Labiatae)

Fresh basil makes a delicious addition to tomato dishes and is also an important ingredient in pesto sauce.

DATA FILE

PLANT DESCRIPTION: Bushy, highly aromatic annual with branched stems (2 ft/60 cm). Oval, dark green, shiny fragrant leaves; white flowers in whorls in midsummer. Several other types of basil exist, including purple ruffled basil, Greek basil, and lemon basil; Indian basil is called Tulsi (*Ocimum sanctum*).

CULTIVATION: Grow from seed under glass in spring, or outside once frost has passed. Needs rich, moist soil with full sun and protection from cold; grows well in pots. For maximum yield of leaves, pinch out the flowers as they appear.

USEFUL PLANT PARTS: Fresh or dried leaves (dried have less flavor).

MAIN USES: Infusion of leaves helps relieve nervous stress, headaches, and nausea; plant acts as an insect repellant. Use basil in the kitchen to make pesto sauce, or with tomato dishes.

Try making an infusion of basil leaves to help relieve stress, headaches, and nausea. You can use fresh or dried leaves.

HISTORY

The name "basil" comes from the Greek "*basileus*" —a king: Parkinson said, "The smell thereof is so excellent that it is fit for a king's house." Strange superstitions in the Mediterranean linked basil to scorpions: Culpeper called it "a herb of Mars and under the Scorpion."

Evening primrose

Oenothera biennis (Onagraceae)

DATA FILE

PLANT DESCRIPTION: A strong perennial plant with thick fleshy roots and narrow willow-like leaves. Tall stems (up to 6 ft/1.8 m) bear large, sweetly fragranced, golden flowers that each last a single day, to be followed by seed capsules.

CULTIVATION: In the wild, it prefers dry, sandy locations; sow seeds in a light, well-drained soil in full sun. The plant is in flower continually from June to fall.

USEFUL PLANT PARTS: Leaves, stems, and flowers (fresh), and roots dug fresh.

MAIN USES: An infusion of the leaves is helpful for colds and flu. Native American healers use the root in poultices for boils or infected skin. The roots can be boiled and eaten as a vegetable. The vegetable oil extracted from the plant is rich in GLA (gamma-linoleic acid) and is taken as a supplement to help PMS, skin problems, and rheumatoid arthritis.

Evening primrose grows in the wild in dry, sandy places such as sand dunes and sandy soil. It also thrives on wasteland. It is native to North America but now grows worldwide.

HISTORY

According to Mrs Grieve, the evening primrose, originally from North America, may have been introduced into Italy and then spread into the rest of Europe. It now grows freely in the wild in Great Britain.

Leaves, stems, flowers, and roots are all used medicinally. The oil has also now become popular for relieving menstrual problems.

Marjoram (sweet)

Origanum marjorana
(Labiatae/Lamiaceae)

Marjoram has a long history of use in cookery and in medicine. It grows in Europe, the Middle East, and North Africa.

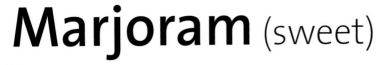

HISTORY

Originally native to the Mediterranean region, marjoram has been used as a medicinal and culinary herb since ancient Egyptian times. It was probably introduced to Britain in the Middle Ages.

Place a few marjoram leaves in a cheesecloth bag to feel the benefit.

DATA FILE

PLANT DESCRIPTION: An attractive herb (up to 10 in/25 cm) with oval, short-stalked, aromatic leaves and white or pinkish flowers on reddish stalks.

CULTIVATION: Although the plant is strictly a perennial, poor frost resistance may mean that it needs to be replanted each year. It is useful as a container herb. Seeds can be planted outdoors in April, in a warm sunny spot with a light rich soil. Containers should be brought indoors in winter.

PLANT PARTS USED: Leaves (fresh or dried slowly in the shade to preserve the aromatic quality). The flowering stems yield an essential oil by distillation.

MAIN USES: As an ointment or in the bath, the leaves and flowers soothe aches and pains and rheumatic joints. Infusion of marjoram helps nervous indigestion and tension. As a flavoring, marjoram is excellent in soups, tomato sauces, and meat dishes.

Oregano

Origanum vulgare
(Labiatae/Lamiaceae)

Oregano is a bushy herb that produces clusters of pink flowers late in the summer.

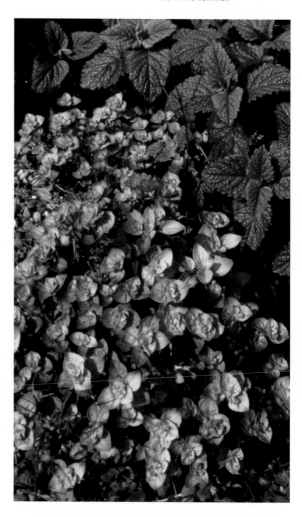

DATA FILE

PLANT DESCRIPTION: Bushy perennial herb with erect reddish stems (up to 30 in/75 cm). Soft, pointed, gray-green leaves are highly aromatic and tiny clusters of pink flowers occur in late summer.

CULTIVATION: Grows wild on dry, chalky hillsides in the Mediterranean; cultivation requires a light, very well-drained soil and full sun to maximize the aroma. Can be sown from seed in spring or root clumps divided. Pinch out flowers for maximum leaf production in summer.

PLANT PARTS USED: Leaves (fresh or dried in shade for full aroma).

MAIN USES: Infused leaves help indigestion, exhaustion, and menstrual pain. In the bath, oregano eases aches and pains and soothes stress. In the kitchen, oregano adds a strong, warm flavor to tomato dishes, pizza, and Greek salad.

The fresh and dried herb is very popular in cookery and adds a tantalizing flavor to pizzas, tomato dishes, and salads.

HISTORY

The name "origanum" comes from two Greek words: *oros* meaning mountain and *ganos* meaning joy; one of its common names is still "joy of the mountain." The Greeks used oregano internally and externally as a remedy, and in medieval times the powerful fragrance made this a useful strewing herb.

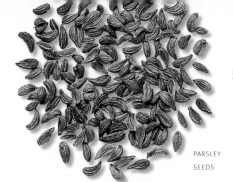

Parsley

Petroselinum crispum (Umbelliferae)

DATA FILE

PLANT DESCRIPTION: A biennial herb with a vertical tap root, tall stems (up to 30 in/75 cm) and tightly curled, rich green leaves. Flat-topped flowerheads with yellowish blooms are followed by capsules with brown seeds.

CULTIVATION: Needs a moist, well-worked soil. Parsley will tolerate some shade. For continuous supplies of leaves, try planting three sowings, in early March, May, and July. In the summer, keep the plants well-watered.

PLANT PARTS USED: Leaves (fresh, or may be frozen) and roots (dug in winter and dried).

MAIN USES: Parsley is a strong diuretic; infusion of the roots or leaves helps urinary infections and fluid retention. It helps the body excrete toxins, which is useful in conditions like gout. The leaves are delicious used in herb butters, soups, and salads as a garnish. Parsley is rich in Vitamin C.

HISTORY

The Greeks used parsley in their funeral rites and considered it to be sacred to Persephone, the Queen of the Underworld. Herbalist John Gerard (see page 13) believed the roots and seeds were a remedy against poison, the seeds being the most active part.

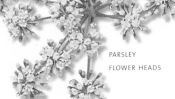

Chopped fresh parsley makes a delicious garnish for soups, salads, and savory bakes.

CAUTION
Do not use medicinally in pregnancy or kidney disease.

Parsley is native to Europe but is grown around the world as a culinary herb. It is rich in vitamin C.

PARSLEY
FLOWER HEADS

Rosemary

Rosmarinus officinalis
(Labiatae/Lamiaceae)

Dried rosemary leaves also have medicinal value and can be used in the same way as fresh leaves.

HISTORY

Used since ancient times as an incense, to decorate places of worship, and as an ingredient in wedding bouquets, symbolizing love and loyalty.

You can use an infusion of rosemary leaves as a tonic for your scalp and hair.

DATA FILE

PLANT DESCRIPTION: Tall, woody, evergreen shrub (up to 10 ft/3 m). Bushy stems with velvety young shoots produce long, narrow, very aromatic leaves, dark green on top and whitish below. The blue flowers are highly attractive to bees.

CULTIVATION: Needs a light, very well-drained soil and a warm sunny position. Grow it from seed, cuttings, or layering (this involves pegging down long shoots close to the ground to encourage rooting.)

PLANT PARTS USED: Leaves (fresh or dried); leaves and shoots used for distillation of the essential oil.

MAIN USES: Infusion of rosemary leaves helps headaches and stress and also may be used as a scalp and hair tonic. An ointment of the leaves is very helpful for aches and pains and rheumatism. In the kitchen, rosemary flavors lamb and other red meats; vegetarians may like it in a nut roast!

CAUTION
Do not drink infusions for more than one week at a time; not recommended during pregnancy.

ROSEMARY

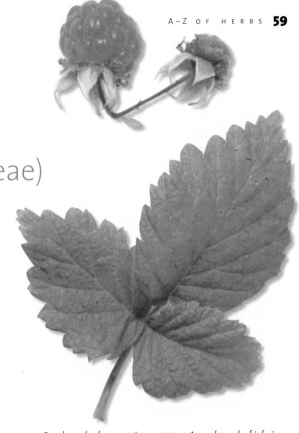

Raspberry

Rubus idaeus (Rosaceae)

DATA FILE

PLANT DESCRIPTION: Deciduous shrub with tall, woody, prickly stems up to (5 ft/1.5 m). The pointed, serrated leaves are arranged in threes or sevens, and are glossy on top and whitish below. White flowers bloom on second year stems, and the fruit is a red compound berry.

CULTIVATION: Requires a well-worked soil with plenty of organic matter. Bushes are usually grown in a row so they form a hedge. They need protection from wind and prefer a slightly acid soil. They will start fruiting in their second year.

PLANT PARTS USED: Leaves (fresh or dried) and fruit (eaten fresh or frozen).

MAIN USES: Infusion of the leaves is a pleasant drink that soothes sore throats or mouth ulcers and eases stomach aches or indigestion. A poultice of the leaves helps to clean cuts or wounds. The fruits are a delicious source of Vitamin C.

ABOVE *Raspberry bushes grow in the wild and are also cultivated in gardens in mild climates. The delicious berries are a valuable source of vitamin C.*

BELOW *A raspberry leaf infusion is excellent for soothing a sore throat. It can also ease mouth ulcers and relieve stomach aches and indigestion.*

HISTORY

Rubus means thorny and *idaeus* refers to Mount Ida in Asia Minor, where the plant grew wild in profusion. Originally a wild shrub, there are now many cultivated varieties available. Traditionally, an infusion of the leaves was said to assist women in childbirth.

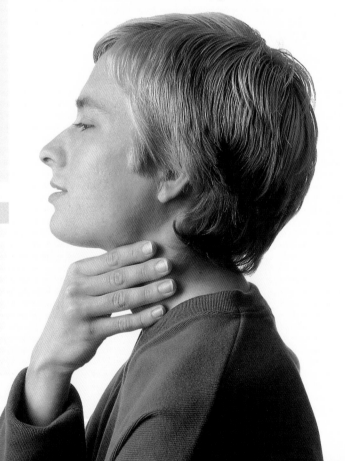

Sorrel (common)

Rumex acetosa (Polygonaceae)

DATA FILE

PLANT DESCRIPTION: Perennial herb (up to 4 ft/ 1.2 m) with juicy stems, large, thick, shiny leaves, and tall spikes of reddish flowers in late summer.

CULTIVATION: Grows wild in damp fields and on waste land; in the garden it likes a damp, rich soil and needs to be well-watered. It can be grown from seed; the leaves can be cropped frequently and the flowers should be pinched out to encourage more leafy growth.

PLANT PARTS USED: Leaves (fresh).

MAIN USES: Infusion of the young leaves is a good spring tonic, cleansing to the whole system, and helps reduce fevers. Sorrel leaves can be eaten sparingly in salads; the flavor is quite bitter.

CAUTION

The leaves contain oxalic acid, which can cause skin sensitivity in some individuals.

HISTORY

In the 18th century, sorrel was considered to be very strengthening to the appetite and cleansing to the liver; eaten in salads, it was said to purify the blood. An old country recipe for sorrel is to mash up fresh leaves into a paste and add a little sugar and vinegar, then serve with cold meats.

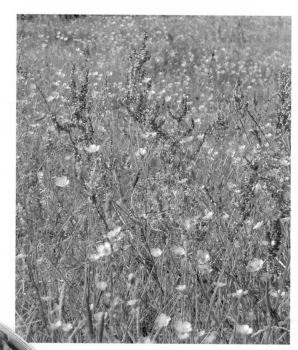

Sorrel grows wild on wasteground and in damp fields. To cultivate it, you will need to use a damp, rich soil and keep it thoroughly watered.

You can add fresh sorrel leaves to salads, but use them sparingly because they are quite bitter.

Sage

Salvia officinalis Labiatae/Lamiaceae

DATA FILE

PLANT DESCRIPTION: Perennial evergreen shrub (up to 30 in/75 cm) with a taproot, square, branching stems, and pointed, gray-green, downy, wrinkled leaves with a strong aroma. Blueish flowers occur in late summer.

CULTIVATION: Needs a well-drained soil and full sun to develop the aroma in the leaves. Grow either from seed or from cuttings. A useful container herb.

PLANT PARTS USED: Leaves (either fresh or dried in shade to preserve the aroma).

MAIN USES: An infusion of sage can help to soothe sore throats, colds, and flu and eases mouth ulcers and sore gums, as well as reducing stress or anxiety. In the kitchen, sage is an excellent flavoring for ham or pork meats, and Mediterranean dishes including pasta; fresh young sage leaves in bread and butter are eaten as a tonic in France.

Sage is a delicious culinary herb and is used to flavor stuffings, as well as meat and poultry.

HISTORY

Originally native to the Mediterranean, with a long history of use as a medicinal and culinary herb. The name salvia comes from the Latin *salvere*, to save. A common French name for it is *toute bonne*, all good.

CAUTION
Do not use medicinally for more than a week at a time because it is a strong herb.

Use a sage infusion to ease the pain of mouth ulcers, sore gums, and sore throats. Sage can also reduce stress and anxiety.

Elder

Sambucus nigra (Caprifoliaceae)

DATA FILE

PLANT DESCRIPTION: Deciduous shrub or small tree with rough, cracked bark and straight branches (up to 30 ft/9 m). Leaves are dull green with 5–7 leaflets; reddish stems bear flat–topped heads of fragrant, creamy flowers followed by shiny black berries.

CULTIVATION: Grows wild in hedgerows or on waste ground; can be cultivated using hardwood cuttings in the fall. It will tolerate partial shade.

USEFUL PLANT PARTS: Flowers, berries (fresh or dried), and young leaves.

MAIN USES: Elderflowers promote sweating; with equal parts of peppermint and yarrow, they make a very effective infusion for colds or flu. The berries have a high vitamin C content and may be made into cordials for coughs and colds, as well as into elderberry wine. The leaves, infused in vegetable oil, are soothing to the skin.

Elderberries are rich in vitamin C and are often made into cordials to soothe coughs and colds. Elderberry wine is an old remedy for sciatica and neuralgia.

Elder is a shrub or small tree that grows wild on wasteland. It produces a profusion of cream-colored flowers and purplish-black berries. The flowers, berries, and leaves are used.

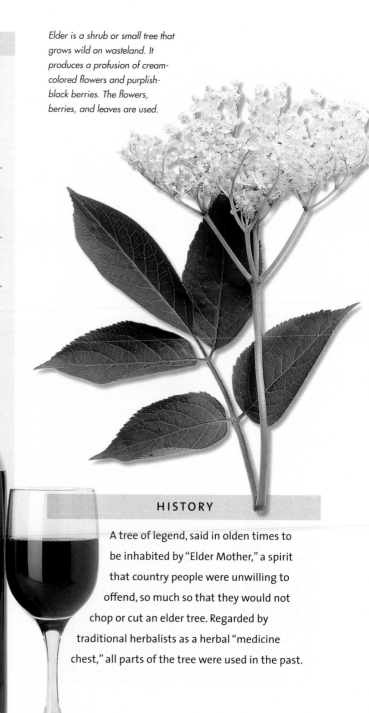

HISTORY

A tree of legend, said in olden times to be inhabited by "Elder Mother," a spirit that country people were unwilling to offend, so much so that they would not chop or cut an elder tree. Regarded by traditional herbalists as a herbal "medicine chest," all parts of the tree were used in the past.

Clover (red)

Trifolium pratense (Leguminosae)

HISTORY

The common name clover comes from the Anglo-Saxon *claefre*. The herb is native to Europe, and is often found growing wild in pastures and fields. It is cultivated as an animal fodder and also ploughed into the soil to enrich it. In the past, red clover has been used as a wound-healer.

This herb can often be found growing wild in pastures and fields in Europe. It is used as animal fodder and to enrich the soil.

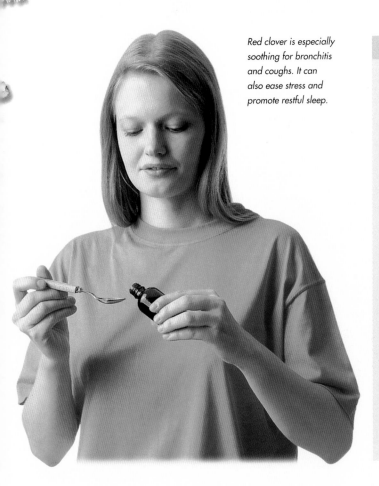

Red clover is especially soothing for bronchitis and coughs. It can also ease stress and promote restful sleep.

DATA FILE

PLANT DESCRIPTION: A short-lived perennial (up to 20 in/50 cm) with branching, slightly hairy stems, and long-stemmed trefoil leaves culminating in fragrant, reddish-purple, dense flower heads.

CULTIVATION: Sow in spring (rub the seeds with fine sandpaper to improve germination) in well-drained, slightly alkaline soil.

USEFUL PLANT PARTS: Flowers and leaves (fresh or gently dried in the dark).

MAIN USES: An infusion of red clover is recommended for bronchitis and coughs. It can also be used as a compress or in the bath to help rashes or sore skin. Infusion of the flowers can reduce stress and help sleep. The young leaves can be added to salads or soups and eaten like spinach.

Thyme

Thymus vulgaris (Labiatae/Lamiaceae)

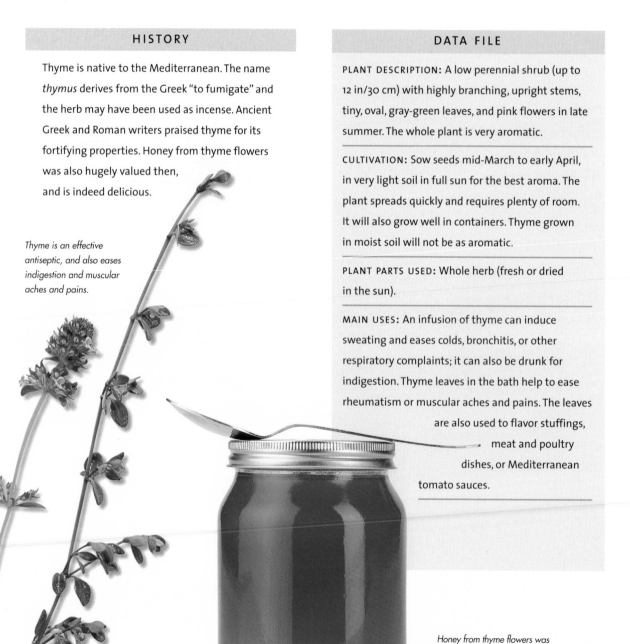

HISTORY

Thyme is native to the Mediterranean. The name *thymus* derives from the Greek "to fumigate" and the herb may have been used as incense. Ancient Greek and Roman writers praised thyme for its fortifying properties. Honey from thyme flowers was also hugely valued then, and is indeed delicious.

Thyme is an effective antiseptic, and also eases indigestion and muscular aches and pains.

DATA FILE

PLANT DESCRIPTION: A low perennial shrub (up to 12 in/30 cm) with highly branching, upright stems, tiny, oval, gray-green leaves, and pink flowers in late summer. The whole plant is very aromatic.

CULTIVATION: Sow seeds mid-March to early April, in very light soil in full sun for the best aroma. The plant spreads quickly and requires plenty of room. It will also grow well in containers. Thyme grown in moist soil will not be as aromatic.

PLANT PARTS USED: Whole herb (fresh or dried in the sun).

MAIN USES: An infusion of thyme can induce sweating and eases colds, bronchitis, or other respiratory complaints; it can also be drunk for indigestion. Thyme leaves in the bath help to ease rheumatism or muscular aches and pains. The leaves are also used to flavor stuffings, meat and poultry dishes, or Mediterranean tomato sauces.

Honey from thyme flowers was prized by the ancient Greeks and Romans. It has a wonderful flavor and is a good source of energy.

Valerian

Valeriana officinalis (Valerianaceae)

DATA FILE

PLANT DESCRIPTION: A perennial herb with a very extensive, strong-smelling root system, and stout hollow stems (up to 4 ft/1.2 m). The leaves are bright green and slightly serrated at the edges, and pinkish-white flowers are produced in clusters in the summer.

CULTIVATION: Valerian requires rich, moist soil and it will tolerate some shade. Established plants need an annual dressing with manure.

PLANT PARTS USED: Roots (must be at least two years old, gathered after leaves fall, used fresh or dried in shade).

MAIN USES: Valerian has a very sedative action and is used in herbal medicine to treat stress, tension insomnia, and migraine, as a tincture or as a decoction of the roots.

The valerian plant grows wild in damp conditions in Europe and Asia. To cultivate it, you will need a rich, moist soil. It can tolerate some shade.

HISTORY

In the past, other names for valerian were All-heal, particularly in medieval times when it was used for epilepsy or nervous anxiety, and Phu, so called by classical herbalists because of its powerful odor. John Gerard (see page 13) used it as an ingredient in "counterpoysons," mixtures of herbs to deal with poisoning.

CAUTION

Valerian should not be used in large doses or for too long; it is best taken medicinally under the supervision of a practitioner.

Use a tincture or decoction of valerian to ease stress and tension, soothe migraine, and promote restful sleep.

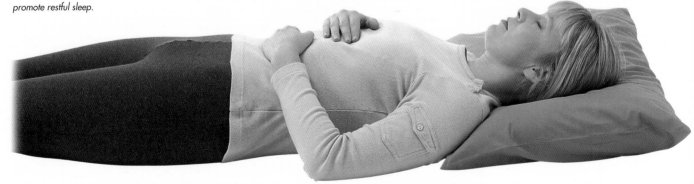

Making herbal preparations

Using herbs on yourself is a wonderful way to gently support your health, easing away everyday aches and pains. The healing properties of herbs can enter the body either through swallowing the plant remedy in liquid form, or by working it in through the skin. These simple methods are very effective and have been used for hundreds of years.

INFUSIONS OR HERBAL TEAS

This is probably the easiest and most convenient way to use herbs. You can, of course, buy herbal teas in sachets, but it is also useful to try herbs you have grown or stored yourself.

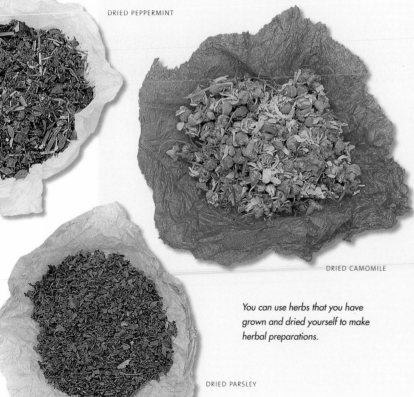

DRIED PEPPERMINT

DRIED CAMOMILE

You can use herbs that you have grown and dried yourself to make herbal preparations.

DRIED PARSLEY

The correct dose is 1 oz/30 g dried herb to 2½ cups/ 600 ml of boiling water. If you are using fresh herbs, you will need twice the amount. Bottled spring water is preferable to tap water.

Place the dried herb in a warmed teapot. Pour over the boiling water and then leave it to infuse for 10–15 minutes.

Teas can be sweetened with honey.

Camomile, fennel, or a mixture like peppermint and melissa all make delicious herbal teas.

Use up the infusion on the day it is made.

Some cooled infusions, such as camomile, also make useful and soothing skin tonics.

MACERATED HERBAL BALMS

These are scented herbal oils that can be rubbed into the skin to condition it or help aches and pains.

You need a heatproof glass bowl that you can place over a saucepan of simmering water.

Half-fill your bowl with clean, washed leaves such as comfrey, and then cover them with a vegetable oil, for example sunflower or grapeseed. Let the oil and leaves sit over the simmering water for about an hour, with a saucepan lid placed gently on top.

At the end of the hour, let the oil mixture cool. Sieve it, then pour it into a bottle and close it tightly. It will last for 4–6 weeks.

Balms made with St John's wort, lavender, rosemary, or elder leaves are very useful for soothing sore skin, burns, and wounds.

You can make a scented herbal oil and rub it into your skin to condition it.

Soothe tired and aching feet by massaging some scented herbal oil into them.

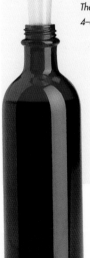

Use a clean funnel to pour the oil mixture into a colored glass bottle. The mixture will keep for 4–6 weeks.

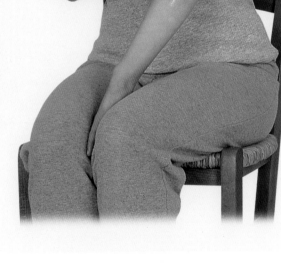

Using herbal oils is also a good way to keep dry skin at bay.

TINCTURES

These mixtures of herbs and alcohol are very potent, so only 30 drops of a tincture are taken in a glass of water once or twice a day.

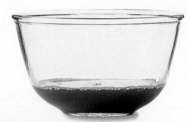

After the herb has steeped in the vodka for two weeks, strain the mixture through cheesecloth into a bowl, then transfer to bottles.

To make a tincture, use 7 oz/200 g herbs to 1¾ pints/1 liter of fluid.

Measure your chosen herb into a large screw-top jar, then cover it with the correct amount of spirit, such as good quality vodka.

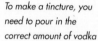

To make a tincture, you need to pour in the correct amount of vodka

Keep it tightly covered in a warm place and shake the jar well twice daily.

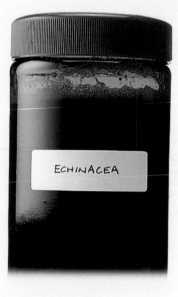

Store your herbal preparations in dark glass jars or bottles until ready for use.

After 14 days, strain the liquid through cheesecloth and into dark glass bottles, keeping them tightly closed.

Plants such as echinacea and oats are used to make tinctures.

ECHINACEA

You can also buy them ready-made from herbalists or health food shops.

USING HERBS

Here are some more interesting ways for using your herbs that require minimal preparation and can be done with the simplest of equipment in your own kitchen.

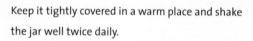

HERBAL BATH BAGS

Make a small drawstring bag out of cheesecloth.

Place in it 3 tablespoons/45 ml oatmeal and several sprigs of fresh herbs, such as lovage leaves, lavender flowers, or rosemary leaves.

Hang the bag over the hot tap so the water runs through it, making the bathwater soft and lightly scented.

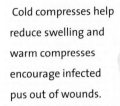

COMPRESSES AND POULTICES

These require you to use clean cloth such as cheesecloth to apply herbs to the skin.

A compress is made by soaking a clean piece of cloth in an infusion and laying it over a burn or a cut and leaving it in place for 10–15 minutes.

Cold compresses help reduce swelling and warm compresses encourage infected pus out of wounds.

For a poultice, gently heat your chosen herb in a little water and mash to a paste, then smear onto the cloth and bind over the affected area.

Calendula or camomile compresses and poultices are helpful for damaged or problem skin.

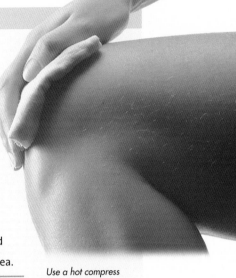

Use a hot compress to expel pus from a wound, and a cold compress to help reduce swelling.

Make a compress by soaking a clean piece of cloth in a herbal infusion. To use it, lay it over the affected part for 10–15 minutes.

SIMPLE OINTMENT

In a heatproof glass bowl, place 5 tablespoons/75 g grated beeswax and 5 tablespoons/75 g cocoa butter.

Add 90 ml/6 tablespoons sweet almond vegetable oil.

Place the bowl over a saucepan of simmering water and stir gently until the waxes and fats combine.

Take the bowl off the heat, and whisking constantly, slowly add 4 tablespoons/60 ml of double strength herbal infusion such as comfrey, calendula, or lavender, beating until the mixture thickens.

Pour into clean, dark glass jars and refrigerate.

Assume a shelf life of two months.

Ointments can be applied to dry skin, cuts, sunburn, and other minor skin problems.

Making your own herbal ointment can be rewarding and satisfying. Remember to label the jars before storing them in the refrigerator.

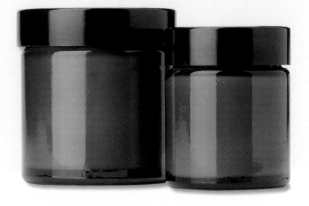

DRIED ROSEMARY

Natural **skin** and **hair** care

In the past, it was common practice to use simple herbal preparations to soothe and condition the skin and hair. Nowadays, most cosmetic preparations are full of synthetic ingredients; if you want to take care of your skin gently and naturally, here are some ideas.

DANDELION AND CAMOMILE FACE MILK

In a heatproof glass bowl, pour ¼ pint/150 ml boiling water on to 3 tablespoons/45 ml each chamomile flowers and chopped dandelion leaves.

Stir well, then cover and leave to steep for 12 hours.

Strain the liquid into another bowl. Add ¼ pint/150 ml of whole cream organic milk and whisk thoroughly. Pour into dark glass bottles and refrigerate.

This milk is a wonderful moisturizing skin cleanser.

Chopped dandelion leaves combined with chamomile flowers produce an excellent face milk.

CALENDULA SKIN TONER

In a heatproof glass bowl, put 8 tablespoons/120 ml calendula petals and flowers.

Pour on 1 pint/568 ml boiling water. Cover and leave for 3–4 hours to infuse.

Strain the liquid, then pour into dark glass bottles and refrigerate.

This toner is an excellent preparation for cleansing the skin of impurities.

This method can also be used with rosemary leaves and the liquid used as a hair–conditioning rinse.

DANDELIONS

MARIGOLD PETALS

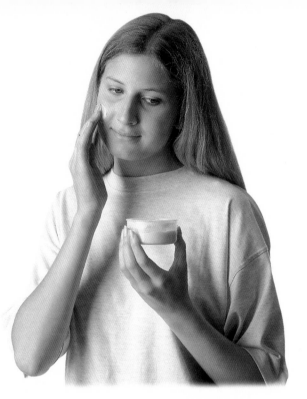

A herbal moisturizer is a gentle, natural way to care for your skin using a variety of pure ingredients to suit your own body's needs.

ELDERFLOWER FACE MOISTURIZER

In a heatproof glass bowl, place three clean, freshly picked sprays of elderflowers.

Pour on 2½ cups/568 ml boiling water, then cover and leave overnight.

In another heatproof glass dish, place 5 tbsps/75 ml sweet almond oil, 1 tbsp/15 ml jojoba oil and 2 tablespoons/30 ml grated beeswax.

Suspend over a saucepan of simmering water, stirring until wax has dissolved.

Remove from heat and then slowly whisk in 4 tbsps/60 ml of the elderflower water until the mixture thickens.

Pour into clean glass jars and refrigerate.

Bottle and use the rest of the elderflower water as a toner or hair rinse.

Elderflowers tone and condition the skin.

SIMPLE HERBAL SHAMPOO

In a heatproof glass bowl place 1 tablespoons/15 ml each of fresh leaves of rosemary, sage, and thyme.

Pour on scant 3 cups/750 ml boiling water and leave to steep for two hours.

Strain the liquid into another bowl, add 4 tablespoons/60 ml good-quality unscented liquid soap, then whisk the two together and pour into dark-colored bottles.

This shampoo tones the scalp and cleans the hair beautifully.

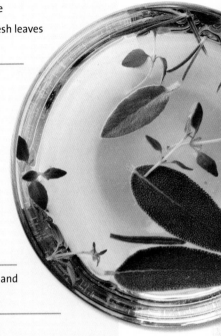

A rosemary, sage, and thyme shampoo will tone your scalp and leave your hair feeling beautifully clean.

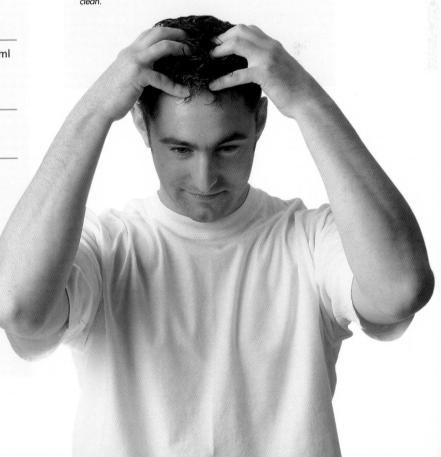

Herbs for general **health care**

Here are some simple suggestions for using herbs to ease common conditions. The ideas here are by no means exhaustive—many of the common herbs can be used: check the A–Z for the best ones to suit you. As has been said before, if you have any serious symptoms, you must consult a professional practitioner.

Herbal infusions, or teas, are an enjoyable way of taking herbs to treat a wide range of ailments.

COUGHS

Elderberry Rob is a pleasant-tasting cough syrup, which can be made up at the end of the summer and stored for use in winter.

Use 5 tablespoons/75 ml ripe elderberries to 1 tablespoon/15 ml dark sugar or apple juice concentrate; the mixture needs to be simmered gently until it is as thick as honey, then cooled, bottled, and stored.

Dissolve 1 tablespoon/15 ml in a mug of very hot water, drunk at night to help clear the chest.

COLDS/FLU

At the first sign of symptoms, make an infusion of yarrow, peppermint, and elderflower combined equally, and drink it hot three or four times a day.

Infused herbs such as sage, thyme, or summer savory are also helpful for colds and flu and can soothe sore throats, especially with a slice of lemon and a spoonful of honey added.

Myrtle leaf tea is also a very good respiratory tonic.

Eat a fresh clove of garlic crushed in your food daily—it boosts your immune system.

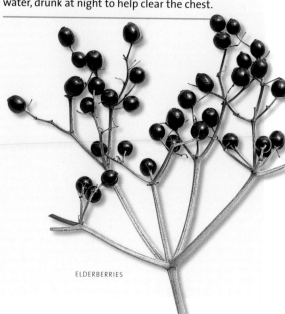

ELDERBERRIES

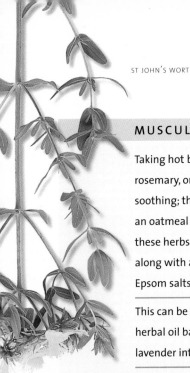

MUSCULAR ACHES

Taking hot baths with thyme, rosemary, or marjoram is wonderfully soothing; the leaves can be placed in an oatmeal bath bag, or an infusion of these herbs can be added to the water, along with a teacupful of sea salt or Epsom salts to envigorate the body.

This can be followed by massaging a herbal oil balm with rosemary and lavender into tired muscles.

St John's wort in a balm massaged into the back eases pain and tension or stiffness.

POOR CIRCULATION

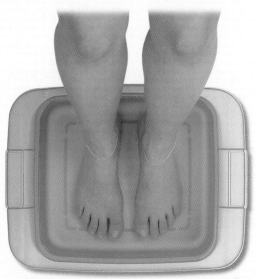

A yarrow or rosemary footbath can ease tired feet and stimulate the circulation.

Massaging a herbal oil balm into the body is an effective way to soothe and invigorate tired muscles and limbs.

Tonics such as angelica, and herbs that increase local blood supply like yarrow or rosemary, can be made into a herbal oil balm and then massaged into the limbs, especially the ankles and feet.

A warm footbath with these herbs can also help poor circulation.

Try including ginger and cayenne in the diet.

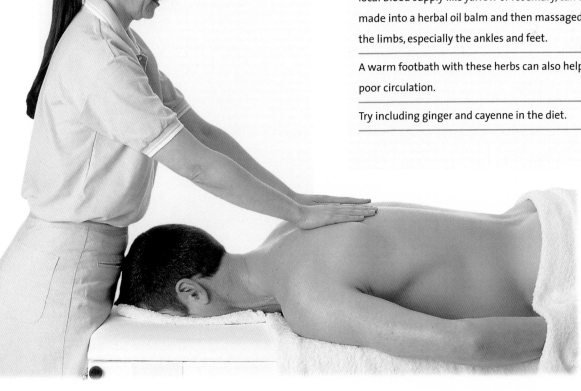

Herbs to **relieve stress**

Modern life is lived at such a fast pace. The conditions on this page are all very closely linked to stress, which is an underlying cause of so many common health concerns. Using herbs is one way to ease stress, but taking time for yourself will also play a big part in managing these symptoms and restoring overall good health.

INDIGESTION

This usually arises through poor eating habits, like rushing food or eating too late at night, or eating foods that disagree with your system.

Eating too quickly, or when stressed or angry, can also bring on indigestion. Bloating, heaviness, dull pain, or heartburn after meals are common symptoms.

As well as considering what and when you are eating, drinking peppermint, fennel, or melissa tea can ease the discomfort and help to settle the stomach.

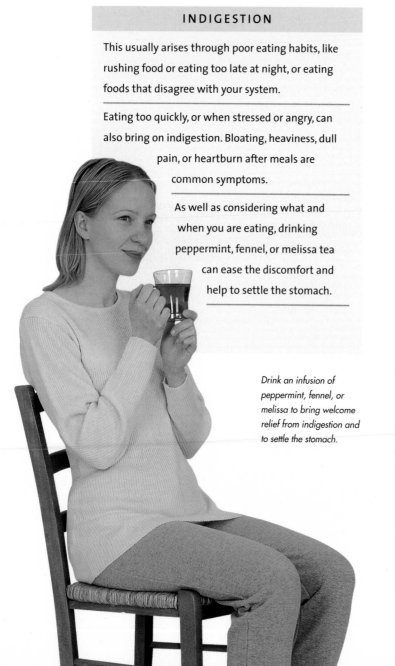

Drink an infusion of peppermint, fennel, or melissa to bring welcome relief from indigestion and to settle the stomach.

INSOMNIA

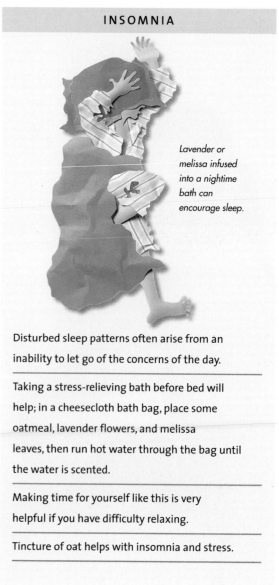

Lavender or melissa infused into a nightime bath can encourage sleep.

Disturbed sleep patterns often arise from an inability to let go of the concerns of the day.

Taking a stress-relieving bath before bed will help; in a cheesecloth bath bag, place some oatmeal, lavender flowers, and melissa leaves, then run hot water through the bag until the water is scented.

Making time for yourself like this is very helpful if you have difficulty relaxing.

Tincture of oat helps with insomnia and stress.

HEADACHES

Frontal headaches around the
eyes may be linked to eye strain;
a cooled camomile infusion
soaked into cotton wool pads
and laid on the eyelids helps to
soothe them. Migraines are
much more severe, with stabbing pains
and distorted vision; in this case
an infusion of feverfew taken
hot two or three times daily is
recommended.

Other useful herbs are
peppermint to help any nausea, or
melissa to calm stress.

A cooled infusion of peppermint and lavender can
be made into a compress. Simply soak a piece of
clean cloth in it and then lay it across the forehead.

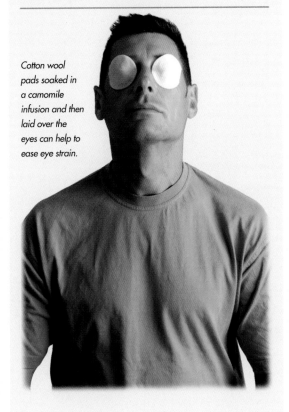

*Cotton wool
pads soaked in
a camomile
infusion and then
laid over the
eyes can help to
ease eye strain.*

EMOTIONAL STRESS AND ANXIETY

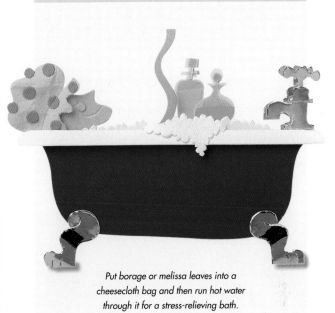

*Put borage or melissa leaves into a
cheesecloth bag and then run hot water
through it for a stress-relieving bath.*

These can potentially deplete your spirits and
depress your immune response.

Try to talk about feelings, release emotional stress,
and take care of yourself above all.

Herbs like borage, melissa,
St John's wort, or rosemary all
help to lift depression; any of
these can be taken as an infusion.

*Lavender flowers are
very restful and soothing
and can help to relieve
stress and anxiety.*

First aid with herbs

The first-aid cabinet can contain several very useful herbal remedies. Contrary to what you might think, herbs can be very swiftly effective as a response to minor injuries. It is best to prepare remedies from herbs you have grown yourself or obtained from a reputable herbal supplier. Some preparations are also commercially available as ointments or tinctures.

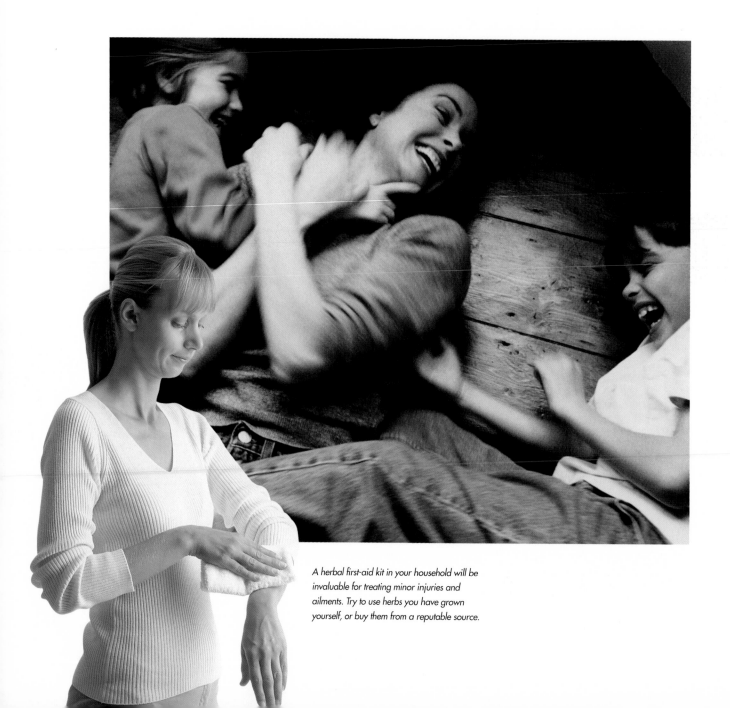

A herbal first-aid kit in your household will be invaluable for treating minor injuries and ailments. Try to use herbs you have grown yourself, or buy them from a reputable source.

DATA FILE

CONDITION	REMEDY AND FIRST—AID METHODS
Sprains	The pain and swelling of torn ligaments requires witch hazel or cool calendula infusion applied as a compress; tincture of arnica given in water to drink for the shock and pain.
Cuts and wounds	Minor cuts can be cleaned with calendula infusion or distilled witch hazel to stop bleeding. For deeper cuts apply pressure, raise the limb, and apply St John's wort applied as a compress or a herbal balm. If bleeding is severe, seek medical help.
Burns	If mild, apply a compress of comfrey infusion followed by comfrey ointment. Aloe vera gel will also help to cool and soothe the skin. Essential oil of lavender (3 drops neat on a gauze pad) is one of the best natural treatments for a burn. Severe burns need medical treatment.
Insect bites and stings	Be aware that allergies to insect bites are becoming more common; any symptoms of collapse or shock need medical help. Simple bites and stings can be soothed with a paste made of sodium bicarbonate mixed with a little water. Aloe vera gel or witch hazel soothe irritation.
Bruising	Cool compresses of witch hazel or comfrey are very helpful. Arnica ointment can be applied immediately if there is no broken skin.
Shock	Symptoms of medical shock are pale, clammy skin, a weak pulse, dizziness, and nausea. Lying the person down and raising the legs, reassuring them, and getting medical help are necessary. Five drops arnica tincture can be sipped in water.

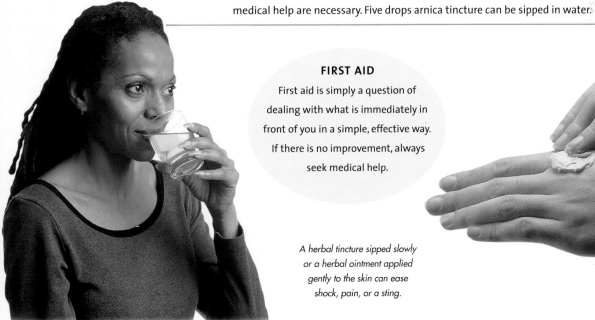

FIRST AID

First aid is simply a question of dealing with what is immediately in front of you in a simple, effective way. If there is no improvement, always seek medical help.

A herbal tincture sipped slowly or a herbal ointment applied gently to the skin can ease shock, pain, or a sting.

Herbs in the **kitchen**

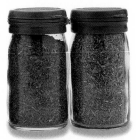

Store dried herbs in jars with tight, well-fitting lids.

Herbs and spices have such a wonderful part to play in flavoring and enhancing all kinds of dishes; used in your food, they also improve your digestive function. Using herbs either fresh or dried from your own garden or balcony is a lovely way to feel you are taking care of yourself as well as making your food more interesting. Here is a simple guide to some common kitchen herbs and spices and their uses.

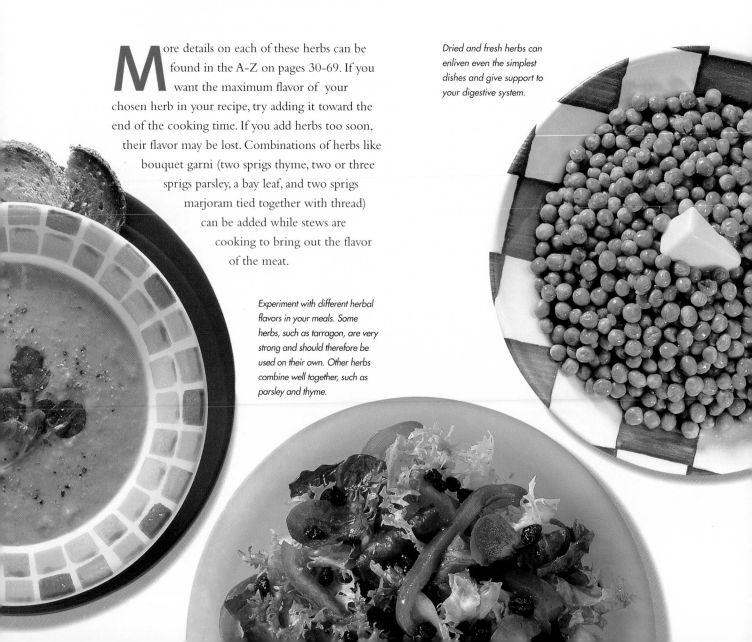

More details on each of these herbs can be found in the A–Z on pages 30–69. If you want the maximum flavor of your chosen herb in your recipe, try adding it toward the end of the cooking time. If you add herbs too soon, their flavor may be lost. Combinations of herbs like bouquet garni (two sprigs thyme, two or three sprigs parsley, a bay leaf, and two sprigs marjoram tied together with thread) can be added while stews are cooking to bring out the flavor of the meat.

Dried and fresh herbs can enliven even the simplest dishes and give support to your digestive system.

Experiment with different herbal flavors in your meals. Some herbs, such as tarragon, are very strong and should therefore be used on their own. Other herbs combine well together, such as parsley and thyme.

DATA FILE

HERB	USES
Basil	fresh or dried leaves in pesto sauce, also with tomato-based Mediterranean dishes
Borage	fresh leaves and flowers in summer wine cups or salads
Chervil	fresh leaves in soups, salads, and egg dishes
Cilantro	fresh leaves in salads and dips with Indian dishes
Fennel	fresh leaves with fish or pork dishes
Garlic	fresh cloves in butter, salad dressings, soups, stews, curries
Lovage	fresh leaves in soups and salads
Marjoram	fresh or dried leaves in meat stews and vegetarian bakes
Parsley	fresh leaves in herb butters, salads, and egg dishes
Peppermint	fresh leaves in mint sauce, or with peas or new potatoes
Oregano	fresh or dried leaves in Greek salad, pizza, or pasta dishes
Rosemary	fresh or dried leaves with lamb and strong meats, or vegetarian nut roast
Sage	fresh or dried leaves with poultry, eggs, or cheese
Savory	fresh or dried leaves with beans, lentils, cabbage, cauliflower, and egg dishes
Tarragon	fresh or dried leaves with poultry, egg dishes, in vinegars and herb butters
Thyme	fresh or dried leaves with tomato sauces and Italian recipes, meats, and cheese

*If you already know the flavors of the
different herbs and the foods they usually
complement, try looking for new
combinations.*

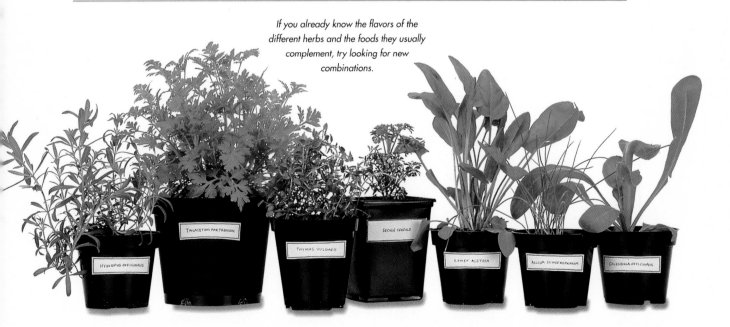

Herbal recipes to enjoy

Here are a few ideas for herbal foods and drinks, flavorings, and garnishes. The more you experiment, you find you will develop your own ways of enhancing recipes. Some of these recipes have been adapted from the cookery books dating back to the early 20th century—it goes to show that our grandmothers had a fine eye for herbs and spices as flavorings in their dishes.

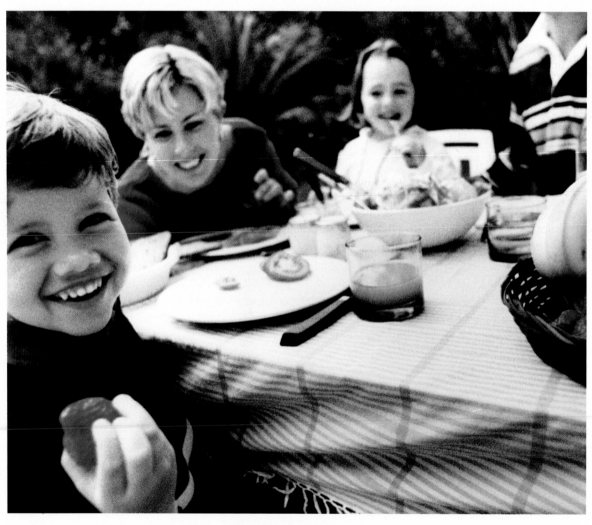

The delicious flavors of herbs can be enjoyed by everyone in your household: try adding them to drinks, sauces, savory dishes, and desserts.

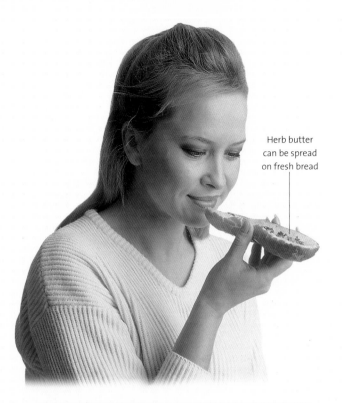

Herb butter
can be spread
on fresh bread

MELISSA CLARET CUP

Pour a bottle of claret or red wine into a bowl, add 2½ cups/568 ml sparkling spring water, four sprigs each melissa and borage, one orange cut into horizontal slices, half a cucumber cut into slices , a small glass of brandy, and 2 tablespoons/ 30 ml dark brown sugar. Leave to sit for an hour before serving.

PESTO SAUCE

In a blender or pestle and mortar, place two cloves crushed garlic, 6 tablespoons/90 ml finely chopped fresh basil leaves, 2 oz/50 g each Parmesan cheese and pine nuts, ¼ pint/ 150 ml virgin olive oil, and sea salt and black pepper, then blend until smooth.

PESTO
SAUCE

HERB BUTTER

To 4 oz/125 g unsalted butter add 1 tablespoon/ 15 ml chopped chives, 2 tablespoons/30 ml chopped parsley, 2 tablespoons/10 ml chopped thyme and chopped marjoram. Beat together and form it into a roll; let cool in the fridge, then cut into slices and serve with soups, bread, or as a garnish for cooked meats.

FRAGRANT, AROMATIC CURRY POWDER

Combine 2 tablespoons/10 ml each ground ginger, ground cardamom, and coriander seed, generous pinch dried cayenne pepper and 2 tablespoons/ 30 ml ground turmeric. Mix together and store in a tightly closed jar. Wonderful for seasoning lentil or vegetable curries.

SORREL SOUP

Gently cook two finely chopped onions and one crushed garlic clove in a little butter. Add two bunches of finely chopped sorrel leaves and stir for a few minutes. Add two medium potatoes, chopped into very small cubes, stir in, then pour on 5 cups/1.2 litres vegetable bouillon. Bring to a boil and simmer for about 15 minutes. The soup can be puréed, then seasoned with salt and pepper, and grated nutmeg sprinkled on top with a swirl of cream to serve.

FRAGRANT
CURRY

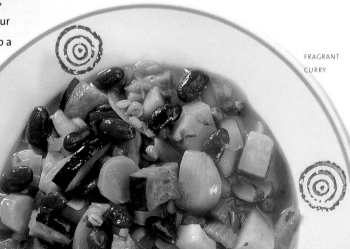

Herbs **around** the **home**

When I was little, I remember quite clearly how my grandmother once dipped her hand into her coat pocket and drew out a handful of lavender flowers for me to smell. She told me that they were used to keep the moths away. I just recall the pleasant flowery fragrance, and the simplicity of the idea. Herbs can be adapted and used very simply to enhance the home.

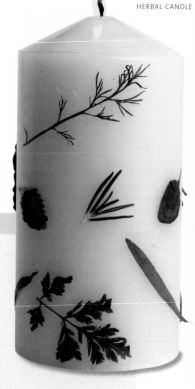

HERBAL CANDLE

POT POURRI

There are different ways of preparing pot pourri, but perhaps the simplest is to use dried ingredients. Pot pourri is a selection of dried scented petals and leaves combined in a bowl, used to fragrance a room. You can be creative with your own mixtures: for a floral aroma, use rose petals, lavender flowers, carnation flowers; for a herbal aroma, you might choose dried rosemary, thyme, marjoram, or sage leaves; for a woody aroma, you could choose sandalwood chippings, myrtle leaves, or pine needles. Combine your chosen ingredients in a plastic bag and leave tightly closed for a week for the aroma to develop, then place in an attractive dish. A few drops of essential oil of one of the plants added to the mixture will maintain the aroma.

HERBAL CANDLES

Fill a tall, heatproof glass jar with boiling water. Hold a large good quality candle in the water by the wick, for about one and a half minutes. Then press flat leaves or petals of favorite flowers into the softened wax. When you have finished, dip the candle back in the boiling water for another minute, and a layer of wax will dissolve over the leaves you have pressed in.

POT POURRI

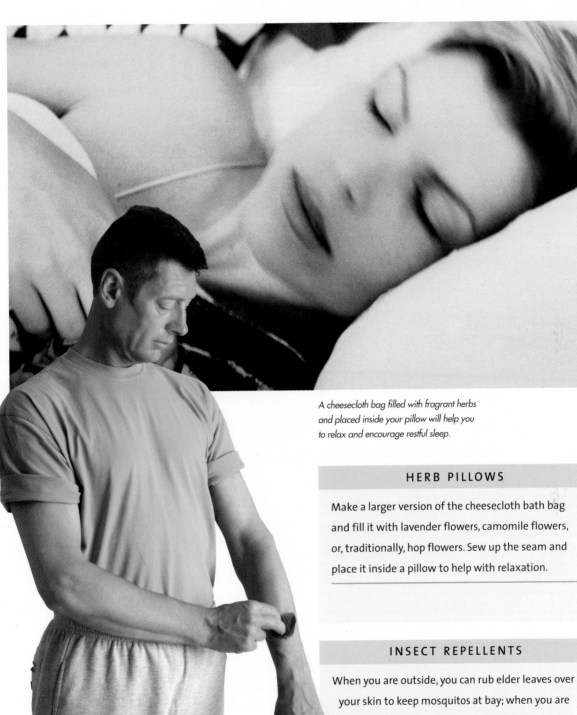

A cheesecloth bag filled with fragrant herbs and placed inside your pillow will help you to relax and encourage restful sleep.

HERB PILLOWS

Make a larger version of the cheesecloth bath bag and fill it with lavender flowers, camomile flowers, or, traditionally, hop flowers. Sew up the seam and place it inside a pillow to help with relaxation.

INSECT REPELLENTS

When you are outside, you can rub elder leaves over your skin to keep mosquitos at bay; when you are indoors, try using candles scented with lavender or citronella essential oils. They make very helpful insect repellants and will ensure your rooms smell delightful.

A medical herbalist—
meet Kelly Holden

No herbal guide would be complete without a contribution from an expert practitioner. Here are some typical questions that people regularly ask Kelly, followed by her own answers, some of which make food for thought! These may answer your questions too.

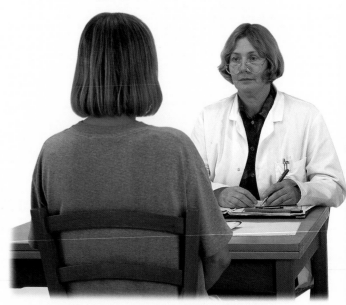

No amount of studying can replace the experience of a qualified practitioner. If you are considering using herbs as medical supports, it is best to receive expert advice.

Q How and why did you become a herbalist?

A I became a herbalist mainly due to my own health challenges. Twenty years ago, I was suffering from a number of different symptoms, including tiredness, headaches, pains in the chest, and numbness, all of which pointed to multiple sclerosis. I read an article in a magazine about a woman who had the same problems and more, who was in fact suffering from mercury poisoning due to the amalgam in her fillings. After reading this, I had my fillings changed, worked with a herbalist and acupuncturist to detoxify my system, and then six months later all my symptoms had gone.

Q Where did you train and for how long?

A Following that experience, my herbalist referred me to the School of Natural Healing run by Kitty Campion, where I went on to train professionally. I did a three-year course by correspondence, weekend modules, thesis, and exams. I qualified in 1985.

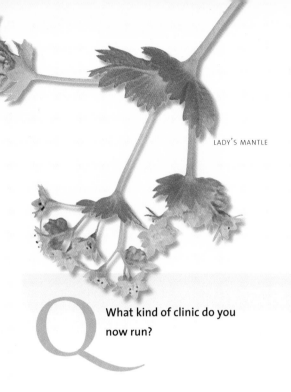

LADY'S MANTLE

Q What kind of clinic do you now run?

A For many years, I ran a practice from home; lately, I have moved with my partner and family and we now have a shop with a house attached which we have converted into a clinic. I am a qualified iridologist, and I practise colonic irrigation and reflexology as well as herbalism. We operate a mail order business alongside the clinic, selling herbal remedies to our clients and to other practitioners.

Q Are there typical conditions patients tend to present you with?

A Yes; low energy seems to underly them all, but I see many clients with Irritable Bowel Syndrome, premenstrual and hormonal problems, menopausal issues, and candida (thrush), also chronic fatigue syndrome (M.E.).

Q Why do patients come for herbal medicine?

A I believe it is because they have lost confidence in conventional medicine. In the UK, about one million people a year consult a herbal practitioner. I think that speaks for itself. However, herbal medicine is not an easy option, and I am very strong with clients—I will not support them in maintaining a lifestyle that is making them sick. If they want results, they have to make changes.

Q Is herbal medicine suitable for children ?

A Absolutely, yes! Children respond very quickly to herbal medicine; their systems have not had time to become so full of toxins. My two sons have never been treated with anything else.

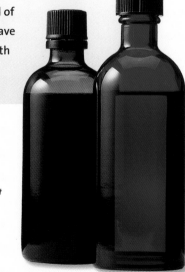

Many people are turning to herbal remedies nowadays because they have lost faith in conventional medicine and want to avoid the side effects often associated with traditional drugs.

Receiving treatment
with herbal medicine

If you are used to Western medicine and doctors, being treated by a herbalist like Kelly is a very different experience. The approach is totally geared toward cleansing your body from the inside out. This may take six months or more: remember you have spent a whole lifetime getting to this point—there is no quick fix.

Before a first consultation, Kelly asks a client to fill in two very detailed questionnaires, one about lifestyle and medical background, and one about yeast-related illnesses such as candida. These questionnaires show the main "challenges," as Kelly likes to call them, and will form the basis of the discussion at the first consultation, lasting three hours. One surprise may be that she is trying to get a picture of the client as a whole, not just simply their immediate symptoms. She will take photos of the iris for iridology purposes, as these can show inherited health patterns. Discussion of the type of cleansing program proposed by her is detailed; she wants the client to appreciate fully the work they will have to undertake. It is a partnership aimed at rebuilding health.

The foundation of any program lies in elimination of years of toxic waste in the system. For at least a month, skin brushing, herbs in capsule form, "superfoods" like spirulina algae, and increased water intake are designed to help the body begin to eliminate more regularly. Only at that point will a specific food program begin, with colonic irrigation to cleanse the bowel. Clients are sometimes surprised that they receive no immediate "prescription" for their stated main complaint; after a few months on the elimination

The detoxification programme includes at least a month of regular skin brushing.

Giving detailed information about your lifestyle and medical background is essential before treatment begins.

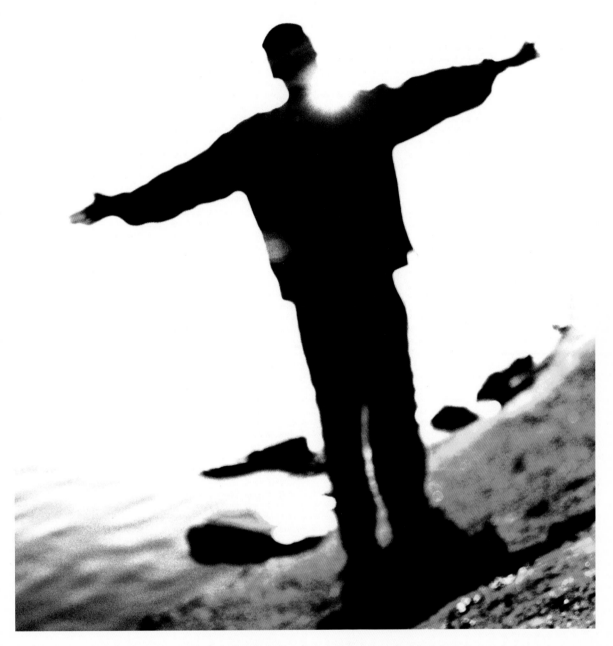

program, they often find their symptoms begin to resolve anyway, as the body cleanses itself. The challenge lies in sticking to the program; follow-up treatments may include reflexology or acupressure to help the process along. Once the body is in a much less toxic state, specific remedies for the main complaint will be used if needed. The aim is to change eating habits to support the system once progress is achieved.

Be patient, it can take a long time to get the body into a more healthy state, but the results can be dramatic.

The difference between this approach and conventional medicine lies in the cleansing of the basic "terrain," the body itself, as the first measure, followed by more specific remedies. It may take six months or more to see improvement, but the effects can be life-changing.

Glossary

ANNUAL: plant that has a one-year life cycle

ASTRINGEROT: a substance that controls tissues and helps stop bleeding

BIENNIAL: plant with a two-year life cycle, flowering and fruiting in the second year

BILE: digestive juice used to break down fats

CULINARY: used in the kitchen

DEADHEADING: pinching out dead flowers in order to encourage new growth

DECIDUOUS: tree or shrub producing leaves in spring and shedding them in fall

DECOCTION: roots or woody plant material boiled in water to obtain active ingredients

DIURETIC: a substance that increases the flow of urine and frequency of passing of urine

DISTILLATION: steam process for evaporating aromas and oils out of plant tissue

EVERGREEN: plant or shrub that does not lose its leaves in winter

GLA (gamma linoteic): fatty acid compound in evening primrose and borage oil, excellent for dry skin

HERBACEOUS: plant which is soft, leafy, and not woody

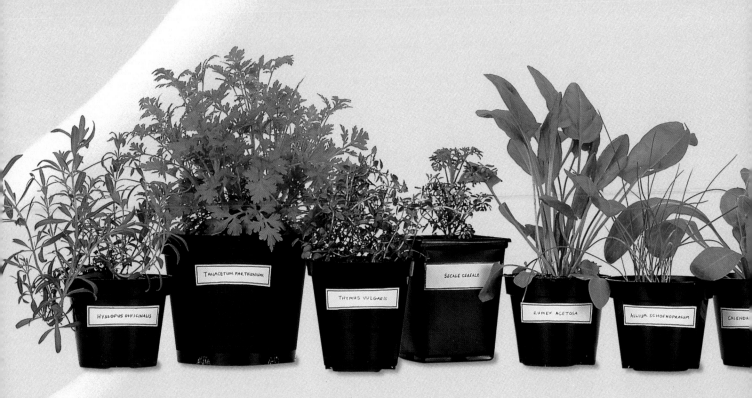

INFUSION: tea made by pouring boiling water on a plant and leaving to sit for 10 minutes

MACERATION: softening of plant tissues by soaking in water or oil

MICROCLIMATE: small area with specific environmental conditions

OINTMENT: fatty base containing plant ingredients with healing properties that is spread on the skin

PERENNIAL: plant living more than two years

PHLEGM mucus coughed up when you have a cold

PROPAGATION: increasing plant supply by taking cuttings, dividing roots, or sowing seeds

RUNNER: a slender creeping stem, which grows along the ground and then takes root to start growing a new plant

STEEPING: leaving herbs to sit in water, alcohol, or oil

TAP ROOT: single large root—for example, dandelion

TINCTURE: herbs or woods preserved in alcohol

TOXIN: poison

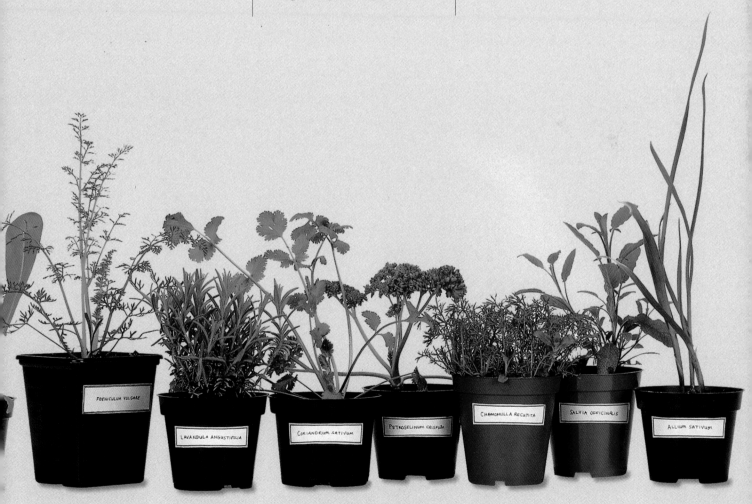

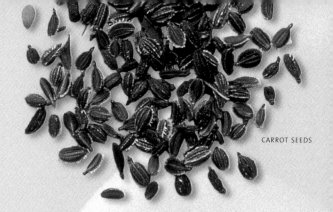

CARROT SEEDS

Useful addresses

HERBAL ORGANISATIONS
You are recommended to contact these bodies for details of qualified practitioners.

UK

British Herbal Medicine Association
Simon Mills
Sun House
Church St
Stroud, Glos, GL5 1JL
Tel: 01453 751389

The Herb Society
Deddington Hill Farm
Warmington
Banbury Oxon
Tel: 01295 692000

USA

American Botanical Council
PO BOX 144345
Austin Texas 78723 USA
Tel: (001) 512 926 4900

USEFUL WEBSITES

UK

www.herbsociety.co.uk
Extensive site with many international links.

www.herbcentre.co.uk Full of information on plants and visitor facilities at the National Herb Centre.

www.botanical.com Extensive site with herbal information and the entire text of Mrs Grieve's 1931 *Herbal*.

USA

www.herbnet.com Huge site with links worldwide.

herbworld@aol.com Site for the Herb Growing and Marketing Network.

www.herbalgram.org Site for the American Botanical Council.

PRACTITIONERS

UK

Kelly Holden
The Holden Natural Health Clinic
The Bield
Lewes Rd
Forest Row
East Sussex RH18 5AF

British Holistic Medical Association
Trust House
Royal Shrewsbury Hospital
Shrewsbury
SY3 8XF

USA

www.christopherhobbs.com
Use site to contact a master herbalist and teacher.

American Holistic Medical Association
Suite 201
4101 Lake Boone Trail
Raleigh
NC 27607

POT POURRI

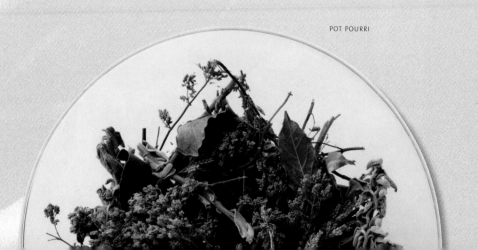

Index

angelica (*Angelica archangelica*) 18, 20, 21, 26, 33, 77

basil (*Ocimum basilicum*) 16, 19, 20, 22, 26, 53, 83, 85
bay tree (*Laurus nobilis*) 19, 22, 47, 82
borage (*Borago officinalis*) 26, 38, 78, 83
burns/scalds 45, 48, 71, 73, 81
calendula (*Calendula officinalis*) 18, 23, 26, 39, 73, 74, 81
carrot (*Daucus carota*) 41, 94
camomile 23, 25, 26, 70, 73, 74, 79, 87
see also Roman camomile
chervil (*Anthriscus cerefolium*) 19, 20, 22, 26, 35, 83
circulation problems 77
clover (*Trifolium pratense*) 67
colds/flu/coughs 30, 33, 38, 46, 51, 52, 54, 61, 62, 63, 67, 68, 76
comfrey (*Symphytum officinale*) 18, 64, 73

coriander/cilantro (*Coriandrum sativum*) 19, 25, 26, 40, 83, 85
culinary uses 82–4
see also flavourings, salad plants

dandelion (*Taraxum officinale*) 26, 65, 74
detoxicants 41, 57, 65
digestion aids 31, 32, 33, 35, 36, 37, 39, 40, 41, 43, 46, 49, 50, 51, 53, 55, 56, 59, 63, 65, 68, 78
diuretics 46, 57, 61, 65
echinacea (*Echinacea angustifolia, E. purpurea*) 42, 72
elder (*Sambucus nigra*) 16, 23, 26, 28, 51, 62, 71, 75, 76, 87
evening primrose (*Oenothera biennis*) 54

fennel (*Foeniculum vulgare*) 19, 22, 25, 26, 43, 70, 78, 83
feverfew (*Tanacetum parthenium*) 18, 23, 26, 66, 79
fevers 34, 60, 66
first aid 36, 42, 44, 45, 48, 52, 59, 73, 80–1
flavorings 35, 36, 40, 43, 47, 49, 50, 51, 53, 55, 56, 58, 61, 63, 68, 82–3

garlic (*Allium sativum*) 19, 26, 32, 76, 83

headache/migraine relief 50, 53, 58, 66, 69, 79

immune system 32, 42, 51, 76
infections 32, 54, 57, 59
insect bites/stings 36, 42, 44, 81
insect repellants 53, 66, 87
insomnia 34, 36, 37, 50, 67, 69, 78, 79, 87

juniper (*Juniperus communis*) 23, 26, 46

lady's mantle (*Alchemilla vulgaris*) 20, 23, 31, 89
lavender (*Lavandula angustifolia*) 16, 19, 20, 22, 23, 26, 28, 48, 71, 73, 79, 81, 86, 87
lovage (*Levisticum officinale*) 18, 20, 21, 22, 26, 49, 83

marigold *see* calendula
marjoram (*Origanum marjorana*) 19, 20, 22, 26, 55, 77, 83, 85, 86
melissa (*Melissa officinalis*) 16, 20, 23, 24, 26, 50, 70, 78, 79, 85

MELISSA

CLOVER

RED SAGE

OATS

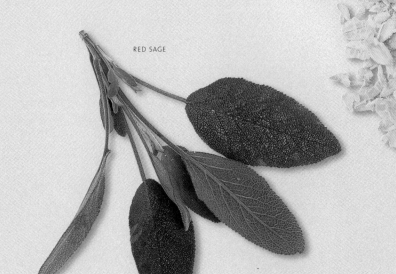

menstrual problems 31, 34, 38, 49, 54, 56
mint 19, 20, 24, 25, 26
see also peppermint
muscular aches 46, 51, 55, 68, 77
myrtle (*Myrtus communis*) 16, 23, 52, 76, 86

oat (*Avenia sativa*) 37, 72, 77, 79
oregano (*Origanum vulgare*) 8, 16, 19, 20, 56, 83

pain relief 55, 58, 59, 68, 71, 77, 79
parsley (*Petroselinum crispum*) 20, 22, 26, 57, 70, 82, 83, 85
peppermint (*Mentha x piperita*) 20, 22, 26, 51, 62, 70, 76, 78, 79, 83

planting and maintenance 24-5

raspberry (*Rubus idaeus*) 59
Roman camomile (*Anthemis nobilis*) 16, 34
rosemary (*Rosmarinus officinalis*) 19, 20, 22, 23, 26, 58, 71, 74, 75, 77, 78, 83, 86

sage (*Salvia officinalis*) 16, 19, 20, 22, 26, 61, 75, 76, 83, 86
St John's wort (*Hypericum perforatum*) 18, 20, 26, 45, 71, 77, 78, 81
salad plants 35, 36, 38, 39, 56, 57, 60, 67, 83
savory (*Satureia hortensis*) 16, 19, 20, 63, 76
skin/hair aids 31, 34, 37, 38, 39, 42, 44, 49, 52, 54, 58, 62, 63, 67, 73, 74-5
sorrel, common (*Rumex acetosa*) 20, 26, 60
stress relief 33, 37, 45, 48, 49, 50, 53, 55, 56, 58, 61, 67, 69, 78-9

tarragon (*Artemisia dracunculus*) 16, 36, 82, 83
thyme (*Thymus vulgaris*) 8, 20, 21, 22, 26, 68, 75, 76, 77, 82, 83, 85, 86
tonics 31, 52, 60, 61, 63, 70, 77
valerian (*Valeriana officinalis*) 18, 20, 69

witch hazel (*Hamamelis virginiana*) 44, 81
wounds 30, 31, 32, 34, 44, 45, 52, 59, 64, 71, 73, 81

yarrow (*Achillea millefolium*) 26, 28, 30, 51, 62, 76, 77

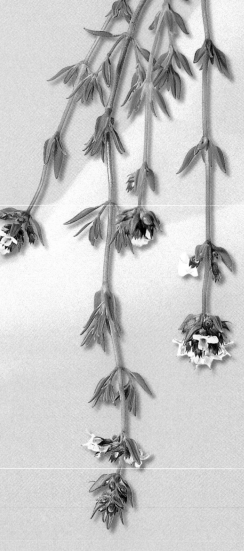

Acknowledgements

Special thanks go to
Jane Lanaway for design and photography co-ordination
Malika Hopkins and Stephanie Winter for help with photography

The publishers would like to thank the following for the use of pictures:
A-Z Botanical Collection 62
Corbis 1 6/7 9 10 15 16 17 18 19L 19TR 20/21 26 28 29 32BL 32R 38 41 48 49 53 55 63 69 87
Harry Smith Collection 36 53
Stone Gettyone 80 84 91
Vanessa Fletcher 8 11 13 54 64
Trudi Valter for picture research